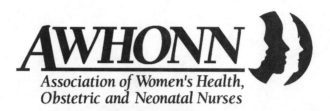

Association of Women's Health, Obstetric and Neonatal Nurses

Single-Room Maternity Care

Planning, Developing, and Operating the 21st Century Maternity System

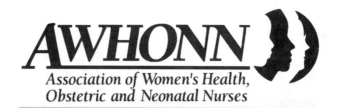

Association of Women's Health, Obstetric and Neonatal Nurses

Single-Room Maternity Care

Planning, Developing, and Operating the 21st Century Maternity System

Celeste R. Phillips, RN, EdD, *1933 -*
President
Phillips + Fenwick
Scotts Valley, California

Loel Fenwick, MD
Chairman
Phillips + Fenwick
Scotts Valley, California

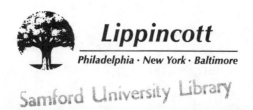

Lippincott
Philadelphia · New York · Baltimore

Acquisitions Editor: Jennifer E. Brogan
Editorial Assistant: Susan Barta Rainey
Senior Project Editor: Tom Gibbons
Senior Production Manager: Helen Ewan
Production Coordinator: Michael Carcel
Design Coordinator: Brett MacNaughton
Manufacturing Manager: William Alberti
Indexer: Michael Ferreira

Library of Congress Cataloging in Publications Data
Phillips, Celeste R., 1933–
   Single room maternity care: planning, developing, and operating
the 21st century maternity system / by Celeste R. Phillips, Loel Fenwick.
     p. cm.
Includes bibliographical references and index.
ISBN 0-7817-2233-0 (paper : alk. paper)
   1. Maternal health services—United States. 2. Postnatal care—United States. 3. Maternal and infant welfare—United States. 4. Hospitals—Maternity services—United States. I. Title: Single room maternity care for the 21st century. II. Fenwick, Loel. III. Association of Women's Health, Obstetric, and Neonatal Nurses.
RG940.P49 2000
362.1′982′00973—dc21

                                   00-023780

Care has been taken to confirm the accuracy of the information presented and to describe generally accepted practices. However, the authors, editors, and publisher are not responsible for errors or omissions or for any consequences from application of the information in this book and make no warranty, express or implied, with respect to the contents of the publication.

The authors, editors and publisher have exerted every effort to ensure that drug selection and dosage set forth in this text are in accordance with current recommendations and practice at the time of publication. However, in view of ongoing research, changes in government regulations, and the constant flow of information relating to drug therapy and drug reactions, the reader is urged to check the package insert for each drug for any change in indications and dosage and for added warnings and precautions. This is particularly important when the recommended agent is a new or infrequently employed drug.

Some drugs and medical devices presented in this publication have Food and Drug Administration (FDA) clearance for limited use in restricted research settings. It is the responsibility of the health care provider to ascertain the FDA status of each drug or device planned for use in their clinical practice.

9 8 7 6 5 4 3 2 1

To
my grandchildren,
Tyler Phillips, Elizabeth Way, Lauren Phillips, and Caroline Way
—Celeste R. Phillips

To
my children,
Bjorn, Stuart, Hannah, and Axel Fenwick
—Loel Fenwick

ABOUT THE
AUTHORS

CELESTE R. PHILLIPS, RN, EdD

Celeste Phillips is president of Phillips+Fenwick, a women's health care development, management, and consulting company based in Santa Cruz County, California. Celeste has an extensive clinical and educational background in maternal-child nursing, including L&D, postpartum, healthy newborn, and prenatal and parenting education. Dr. Phillips has played an active role in defining, teaching, and implementing family-centered maternity care and has actively supported professional organizations, including the Association of Women's Health, Obstetric and Neonatal Nurses (AWHONN) and the International Childbirth Education Association (ICEA). She has helped more than 500 hospitals in the past 20 years to implement contemporary maternity care practices and systems. Celeste has written or coauthored many books, monographs, and journal articles about family-centered maternity care. Her books include *Family-Centered Maternal/Newborn Care; Fathering: Participation in Labor and Birth; Birthing Rooms: Concept and Reality; Family-Centered Maternity Care: Implementation Strategies;* and *Shared Childbirth: A Guide to Family Centered Birth Centers.*

LOEL FENWICK, MD

Loel Fenwick created the Single-Room Maternity Care (SRMC) program and facility as a model for contemporary American maternity care. He invented and developed the modern birthing bed and other equipment and processes for SRMC. Dr. Fenwick has played a part in developing and implementing more than 100 contemporary maternity programs. While practicing as an obstetrician and gynecologist in Spokane, he served as Executive Director for the Cybele Society and served on the board of ASPO Lamaze. He is a writer and speaker on contemporary obstetric practices and programs and has a special interest in family development.

PREFACE

It is more than 20 years since we developed the concept of Single-Room Maternity Care (SRMC). Since its introduction, SRMC has been a model for providing socially responsible maternity care that is aimed at strengthening the family, and with it our future society. SRMC has helped to stimulate a period of profound change in maternity care. Almost every maternity facility today has changed its facilities and practices to make childbearing safer, more comfortable, and more satisfying to families. The idea of family-centered maternity care has been universally embraced, and in many organizations maternity care has risen from underdog status to become the marketing star.

However, there is still considerable confusion about what SRMC is. SRMC is a program of care. It is more than a facility design, more than customer service, more than a marketing program. It is a comprehensive, socially responsible approach to improving family beginnings, family by family. The SRMC program begins before conception and continues through the childbearing year. It is built upon new attitudes and new skills. SRMC challenges family care professionals at all levels to take on a more important role in family development. Along with these challenges, it brings rewards greater than anything that we have experienced before.

Twenty years after its introduction, few American hospitals have functional SRMC programs. In spite of the advantages of the SRMC program of care, relatively few hospitals have been able to successfully implement a comprehensive SRMC program. This is not because the SRMC program is difficult to operate. The effectiveness of the program has been validated by the long-term experience of many facilities that have found SRMC to be highly functional and also preferred by maternity providers and nursing staff. In our experience, the primary reason is that SRMC is an entirely new program that requires an entirely new approach to care to make it work. SRMC generally cannot be achieved by modifying existing multitransfer programs.

SRMC is different from the multitransfer system in which generations of doctors and nurses have trained and practiced. The SRMC program has a different philosophy, goal, clinical practice, and relationship between providers, nurses, and families. Every person who makes an SRMC program work—doctor, nurse, midwife, manager—must move on from familiar and comfortable values and behaviors to learn and practice new clinical and interpersonal skills. Taken together, these differences add up to a major change in an organization's culture and behavior.

An organization's culture, like an individual's personality, is innately resistant to change. Organizations rarely alter their cultures from within, even when many of its members wish for something different. It takes a strong external influence—a major change in the organization's environment or strong new leadership—to re-form long-held beliefs and practices. Few hospitals have been willing or able to make the philosophical changes and learn the new skills required for successful implementation of SRMC programs. The result is that most of America's maternity services are in transition between the old multitransfer surgical system and contemporary models of care.

- Philosophy of care is in transition. The belief that childbirth is a medical/ surgical procedure to be performed upon a patient is giving way to a view that childbirth is a biological and psychological milestone in a woman's and her family's development.
- The goals of maternity care are in transition. Maternal and fetal morbidity and mortality are no longer the only yardsticks by which quality of care is measured. Today, most maternity facilities also want families to be satisfied with their care. Beyond that, some see a professional opportunity and responsibility to support new family beginnings.
- Medical practice is in transition. Instead of following rigid routines passed down from the 1960s, many doctors have individualized their care to match the mother's needs and support her capabilities.
- Maternity nursing is in transition. Where once maternity nurses functioned in a subspecialty of labor and delivery, postpartum or newborn care, many have developed core skills in all aspects of maternity care.
- Newborn care is in transition. Where once care for mothers and babies was fragmented into separate departments and separate patients were cared for by separate medical and nursing staff, mother–baby care provides comprehensive care for mother and baby together.
- Maternity facilities are in transition. Multitransfer systems are being modified by the addition of LDR rooms; others are being replaced by SRMC facilities designed to keep the family together in the same room (LDRP) throughout their maternity stay.
- The maternity service is in transition. Where obstetrics was once regarded and operated as just another surgical service, hospitals are recognizing the special importance of serving families and have implemented family-centered maternity care.

An SRMC program represents the completed passage through these transitions. In the pages to come, we will describe the philosophy that drives SRMC, the programs that make it succeed, and detail how each new element fits into the overall program and supports the goal of strengthening family beginnings.

It is beyond the scope of any book to teach all that has to be known to implement an SRMC program, and this book does not attempt to do so. Instead, its goal is to provide an understanding of what SRMC is all about—what it is, why it exists, how it works, what it takes, what it gives, what makes it succeed, what makes it fail. From this, we hope that the reader will be able to approach implementation of a SRMC program with knowledge and confidence and avoid the missteps that have been made by so many others. Most of all, we hope that she or he will recognize the enormous power for good that is the potential of SRMC, and take up the challenge of using his or her professional skills in a new way to support better family beginnings.

ACKNOWLEDGMENTS

We want to thank the following colleagues for reviewing or contributing to this book:

Bonnie L. Anderson, BS, RN, LCCE, FACCE; Nina Clymer, RN, MBA; Kathy Etherton, BS; Cynthia Fitzgerald, MSN, ARNP; Elizabeth Hamilton, PhD: Diane Himwich, RN, MS, CNAA; Linda K. Todd, MPH, ICCE; Tim Ward, PhD; Henry E. Wells, CPA, FHFMA, DABFA; and Jack Wirnowski, BS, MBA. Their experience and expertise in Single-Room Maternity Care planning, development, and operation was invaluable in the writing of this book.

Of course, this book couldn't have been written at all without all the childbearing families we have known over the years and the SRMC program staffs and leaders with whom we have worked. In addition, special thanks go to the hospitals that participated in the survey we used for this book.

Landis Gwynn, Shirley Coe, Henci Goer, Susan Pease, and Amy Neiblum were extremely patient with our writing and rewriting. And perhaps the most patient and understanding of our need to write this book were our respective spouses: Roger Phillips and Olson Fenwick.

We thank them all.

CONTENTS

CHAPTER 5

CHAPTER 6

CHAPTER 7

CHAPTER 8

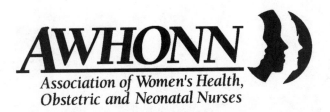

AWHONN
Association of Women's Health,
Obstetric and Neonatal Nurses

Single-Room
Maternity Care

Planning, Developing,
and Operating the 21st Century
Maternity System

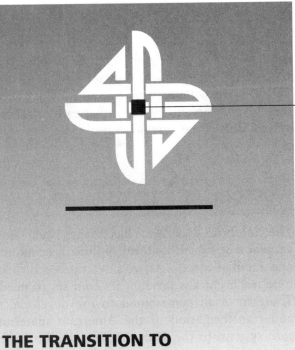

CHAPTER 1

What Business Are We In?

THE TRANSITION TO PARENTHOOD

Why is each woman's memory of every childbirth so clear? Why is it that women do not forget the day, the hour, the moment of their child's birth? Why is it that long past a time when an old woman has forgotten details of weddings, funerals, or holidays, she can recall with clarity the events of each of her children's births? Why is it that families do not discuss childbirth in the factual way they might talk about an illness or surgery? It is because childbirth is both a physical and an emotional event with the power to transform. Having come through the experience of childbirth, we are fundamentally different people than we were before we entered it. Even those among us who most desire to remain un-changed, to not lose ourselves in the experience of childbirth, will be radically altered by it. The birth of each child changes each participant, the family into which that child was born, and the social group in which the family participates.

Becoming a parent is a transforming event. More than any other milestone in life—more than one's birth, graduation, religious or tribal initiation—childbirth is the defining event that marks a man's and woman's transition from the freedom of adolescence to the responsibilities of adulthood. Young adults must shift their attention from their own needs to include the needs of a new human being who is absolutely dependent on them. Then the new parents must successfully raise their young through a critical formative period that will challenge the parents' skills, resources, and patience. If a mother and father fail to form a nurturing family, the results can be disastrous for their children. If many parents fail, the results can be disastrous for the community and society at large.

The transition to parenthood has multiple components. The most basic of these is biological reproduction—the physical elements of pregnancy, birth, and newborn care. However, birth contributes more than just a new family member. It is a personal landmark—an enormous personal accomplishment and a potential source of self-confidence and self-esteem.

Every society recognizes that new parents must have means, skills, confidence, and support if they are to raise their children successfully. Since earliest times, almost every culture has surrounded pregnancy, childbirth, and the newborn period with special care and support (Kay, 1982). Preparation for parenthood was woven into the everyday fabric of community upbringing. Raising a new generation of citizens was understood to be the central purpose of sex and marriage, and this connection was ritualized in ceremony and maintained in custom and expectation. In bringing a new member into the community, parents drew upon community wisdom and support (Kay, 1982). Certainly, there was a time when it took a village to raise a child. In today's self-absorbed and insular lifestyle, those days are long gone. Now, with widespread family dysfunction extracting an incalculable toll on our society, there is a need to make whole again the societal support system necessary for launching each new family.

As healthcare providers, why is this important to us? Those of us who interact with families during pregnancy, childbirth, and newborn care have a unique advantage over anyone else, over any government agency, in helping new parents to succeed. Not only does our contact take place when the parents experience their greatest need for guidance and support, it also coincides with an especially sensitive period during which the pregnant couple have an intense interest in their pregnancy (Colman & Colman, 1971) and what it means to their lives.

Most couples start off with almost no idea how childbirth and parenting will change their futures; consequently, they do not plan for these changes. Even when a pregnancy is confirmed, most couples feel no compelling urge to change the priorities that guide their lives. Women's psychological responses progress during pregnancy from uncertainty and ambivalence to feelings of vulnerability and preparation for the infant's birth (Rubin, 1970; Rubin, 1975). Pregnancy is a time of dramatic emotional swings for both mother- and father-to-be.

In the second trimester of pregnancy, fetal movement announces the undeniable reality of a new presence. This can be a dramatic event to the woman, marking the beginning of the precious "sensitive period" during which pregnant women are more willing than at any other time to focus attention on the needs of their child and future family (Rubin, 1975). This period of heightened awareness and receptivity may be different for fathers, who have a time lag in "knowing" that the pregnancy is real. The most powerful reality boosters for the expectant father during pregnancy are hearing the fetal heartbeat, feeling the fetus move, and viewing the infant on a sonogram (May, 1982; Phillips & Anzalone, 1982).

The childbearing year—the approximately year-long association of interested, needful, focused parents-to-be and healthcare professionals—represents a golden opportunity to support family beginnings. Although supporting the family is important at any time, seldom is there as good an opportunity as during the childbearing year to have close and frequent contact with both parents. As we will see, this opportunity has been largely overlooked by the American healthcare system during the past 60 years.

HISTORICAL BACKGROUND

The childbirth experience has always been a convergence of social, cultural, political, economic, and familial forces. As we have moved through time, each era has brought its own set of needs. These have all contributed to the development and transformation of the American maternity care system. In the 19th century, childbirth was accepted as part of the normal life cycle, usually occurring at home. Women enjoyed special respect and attention as they gave birth in their own homes, supported by family and friends.

Home to Hospital Era

The shift from home birth to hospital birth is a 20th-century phenomenon. Within little more than 100 years, childbirth in the United States was transformed from a normal life event attended mostly by midwives in women's homes to a medical procedure attended by obstetric specialists in hospitals (Wertz & Wertz, 1989).

In 1900, less than 5 percent of all American babies were born in hospitals; by 1940 the figure had increased to 50 percent. By 1970, approximately 99 percent of births occurred in hospitals (Wertz & Wertz, 1989), a percentage that continues to this very day (Rooks, 1997). A number of factors fueled this dramatic change.

First was a belief that hospital births were safer for both mother and baby. Another factor was the availability of analgesia and anesthesia for childbirth in a hospital. The scarcity of hired help after World War I also made the hospital desirable as a place to recuperate after childbirth (Wertz & Wertz, 1989). During the 1920s and 1930s, hospital births attended by a male physician and with anesthesia became fashionable. Home birth with a midwife came to be seen as the province of poor women who could not afford "the best." The baby boom, coupled with a shortage of physicians and nurses after World War II, made institutionalization for birth efficient and preferable for most people. Finally, with the development of third-party reimbursement, medical insurance paid for hospital births but seldom for home births.

However, hospital birth in those early years was not without problems and high infection rates. The uncontrolled and inappropriate use of interventions contributed to unacceptable maternal and infant mortality rates (Speert, 1980). Indeed, in the early 20th century these rates were often higher in hospitals than at home (Porges, 1985).

In response to this, concerned practitioners addressed the misuse of interventions through better training and oversight, and hospital staffs adopted a number of strategies to address infection control. These measures affected hospital policies and facility design. Labor and delivery suites were designed to mimic surgical operating rooms with "vitrified tile floors" and with all deliveries performed on an operating table (DeLee, 1927) (Figure 1-1). All deliveries, it should be noted, were

operative deliveries involving general anesthesia, large episiotomies, and forceps extractions. This was due to a belief in the innate pathology of the natural process and the innate inadequacy of women to give birth (DeLee, 1927).

To combat epidemics of newborn diarrhea and respiratory infections, all babies were sent to hospital nurseries, which practiced strict isolation techniques (DeLee, 1927) (Figure 1-2). Procedures were developed to sterilize rooms, equipment, and beds. Policies restricted visitation and participation of families and friends, who were seen as sources of potential infection (Leavitt, 1989).

The hospital design that resulted was based on the surgical transfer system and used a series of rooms to cater to the series of events that occurred during a mother's hospital stay (Figure 1-3). Most mothers could expect that they and their babies would be cared for in:

1. A preparation room where admission procedures were performed, which routinely included shaving the pubic hair and giving an enema

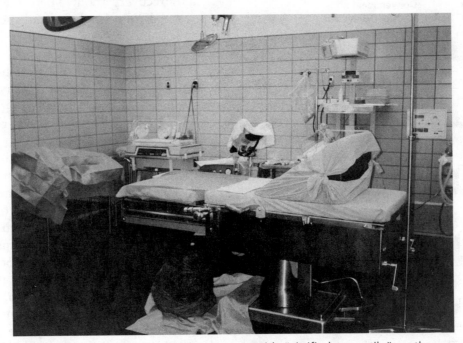

FIGURE 1–1. Conventional delivery room with "vitrified green tile" on the walls.

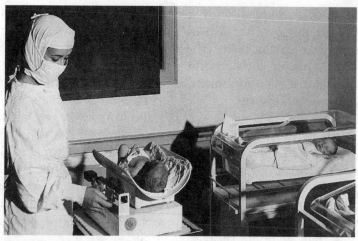

FIGURE 1–2. Traditional newborn nursery where babies were separated from their mothers in an effort to provide "aseptic care."

2. A labor room where women labored alone, often heavily sedated and usually confined to a stretcher or conventional hospital bed, one not well-suited for either labor or delivery
3. An operative delivery room, to which they were transferred for the birth itself; it contained a delivery table designed so that the woman delivered her baby lying prone with her legs suspended in supports, her lower body covered with sterile drapes, and her arms strapped to the delivery table
4. A nursery, to which the baby was routinely sent after birth regardless of the need for any special care; the baby would be brought to the mother for limited periods at scheduled feeding times
5. A recovery room where the mother, separated from her baby and the baby's father, remained for a time after delivery
6. A postpartum ward, to which new mothers were transferred by stretcher and where they remained for 7 to 10 days even with an uncomplicated vaginal delivery; the first 1 to 2 days were spent at bed rest

The view of mother and baby as separate "patients," combined with a sincere effort to prevent infections in both mother and baby, were responsible for the development of the complex system just described that required several different rooms, numerous patient transfers, multiple changes of bedclothes and additional housekeeping, and the need to coordinate the transfer of information among labor room, nursery, and postpartum department personnel. The result was an impersonal, assembly-line experience for the mother, separation for the baby, and exclusion for the father.

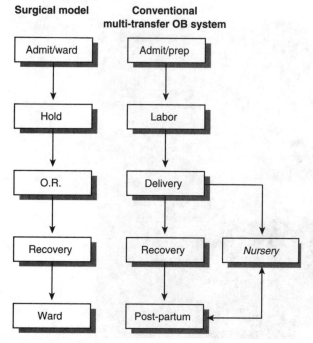

FIGURE 1–3. The system developed for hospital birth was based upon the surgical transfer system.

Nursing care in the separate and distinct facility areas of a maternity service became highly specialized, with some nurses caring only for laboring women, others caring only for postpartum women, others caring for newborn babies, and, later in our history, others caring for sick babies. This meant that maternity services comprised three or four nursing subspecialties operating under two medical departments (obstetrics and pediatrics). One positive result of this fragmentation of nursing care was that nurses within each subspecialty became experts in that area of care. However, a negative result was that no single nurse had an overall understanding of the woman or her family's childbearing experience or the care needs evolving from that experience. The divided staff frequently functioned as if they were in separate departments and worked without the collaboration so important to continuity of family care. This situation often resulted in inefficient care delivery, redundancies, extra tasks, missed communication, mixed messages, and fragmentation in care.

Improvement in Maternal and Child Health

By the middle decades of the 20th century, there were improvements in public health, nutrition, and sanitation (Phillips, 1996). The medical specialty of obstetrics and gynecology became refined and organized (Speert, 1980) and set criteria for hospital safety. As a result, maternal and infant morbidity and mortality statistics improved.

The Awake and Aware Era

As the "baby boom" began after World War II, so did an interest in natural childbirth and childbirth education. In the 1950s, feelings of alienation toward hospital birth began to surface. Although many women had acceptable birth experiences, others bitterly complained about rigid hospital routines, insensitivity—even cruelty—and separation from their babies and families at this important time in their lives (Shultz, 1958). Women and their partners started asking for a better way to give birth and actively pursued alternatives to the conventional, rigid obstetric routines.

Times of Change

Grantly Dick-Read, an English obstetrician, began to teach and speak on the subject of natural childbirth. Dr. Read made a significant contribution by explaining that birth could be an exhilarating experience for a woman and by demonstrating a way in which this could be achieved (Dick-Read, 1953). Prior to the publication of Dick-Read's book, *Childbirth Without Fear,* there was little mention in obstetrics texts about the influence of emotions on labor. Women who had been searching for a better way of giving birth eagerly read his theory on the "fear–tension–pain syndrome," which explained that the discomforts of normal labor can be worsened by the effects of fear and tension. Women began preparing themselves, using Dick-Read's methods, and found that their pain was relieved and birth was a rewarding experience again.

In the 1960s, organized vocal opposition to standard obstetric practice grew. The women's movement contributed to consumer awareness and demand, with consumer organizations advocating for family-centered maternity care (FCMC). Dick-Read's work became the foundation for the first organized programs for family-centered childbirth as well as teacher training. The first of such groups to organize was the International Childbirth Education Association (ICEA), founded in 1960.

At about the same time, the Lamaze method, also known as psychoprophylaxis (PPM), was gaining popularity in the United States due to Elisabeth Bing's leadership. In 1960, the American Society for Psychoprophylaxis in Obstetrics (ASPO) was formed in New York as a national organization to promote the use of the Lamaze method and to prepare teachers of the method (Phillips, 1996).

A Denver obstetrician, Dr. Robert Bradley, published *Husband-Coached Childbirth* in 1965. In this book, he advocated what he proposed as the true natural childbirth, without any form of anesthesia or analgesia and with a "husband-coach" and breathing techniques for labor and birth (Bradley, 1981). The American Academy of Husband-Coached Childbirth (AAHCC) was founded to make the Bradley method available and to prepare teachers.

Ernestine Wiedenbach, a certified nurse midwife, published a text titled *Family-Centered Maternity Nursing* in 1959. In it she wrote of keeping the family together as a unit as much as possible. Wiedenbach described "rooming-in" as an approach that "implies a special attitude toward maternal and infant care, and entails a general plan of supportive maternity care which is based on the recognition and understanding of the needs of each mother, father, infant, and family. Through it, a normal mother-father-infant relationship is encouraged and strengthened" (Wiedenbach, 1959).

When serving as co-presidents of ICEA, Doris and John Haire authored the manual *Implementing Family-Centered Maternity Care with a Central Nursery* (1968) in which they proposed family-centered maternity care to strengthen the new family unit. Their interest in family-centered care was sparked by difficulties they encountered in finding an environment in which they could share a meaningful childbirth experience.

In 1978 a joint position statement on the development of family-centered maternity/newborn care in hospitals was published. This document was the result of collaboration between the major professional organizations responsible for maternal and newborn care: the American College of Obstetricians and Gynecologists, the American College of Nurse-Midwives, the American Academy of Pediatrics, the American Nurses' Association, and the Nurses Association of the American College of Obstetricians and Gynecologists. Key concepts found in the joint position statement are listed in Box 1-1.

During the 1970s, prominent members of the social sciences community and medical, nursing, and midwifery professions were calling for reform of maternal and newborn care. Obstetricians, family practice physicians, sociologists, anthropologists, pediatricians, psychiatrists, midwives, nurses, and other professionals made compelling arguments that there had been a disruption of the core values that were necessary to guide family beginnings.

Two leaders were Drs. Marshall Klaus and John Kennel (1982), who made us aware of the

B O X   1 – 1

Key Concepts of the Joint Position Statement

Key concepts of the 1978 Joint Statement on Family-Centered Maternity Care (FCMC) include:

- The family is the basic unit of society.
- The family is viewed as a whole in which each member is an individual enjoying recognition and entitled to consideration.
- Childbearing and childrearing are unique and important functions of the family.
- Childbearing is a unique experience during which family members benefit from the support of the family unit.
- Integration and bonding of the new family is a high priority.
- Childbearing is a developmental opportunity and/or a situational crisis during which family members benefit from the supporting solidarity of a family unit.

complexity and necessity of mother–baby interaction and what infants needed, as well as what mothers and infants, together, needed. Dr. T. Berry Brazelton's work on the parent–infant interaction experience helped us understand the early parenting experience (Ewy & Youmans, 1988). Dr. Loel Fenwick (Fenwick & Simkin, 1987) wrote about how to return women's biologic capabilities to them and promoted the concept of physiologic birth as a mechanism to improve safety and help women develop self-confidence. Dr. Murray Enkin spoke out for childbearing women and helped launch *Birth and The Family Journal,* publishing articles of the best evidence in opposition to the status quo (Sakala & Swenson, 1999).

Reva Rubin, a nurse educator, wrote about the psychological or emotional experience of childbirth and attainment of the maternal role (Nichols & Humenick, 1988). Celeste Phillips, a maternity nurse educator, published and lectured extensively on father participation in labor and birth (Phillips & Anzalone, 1978). Sheila Kitzinger, a social anthropologist and childbirth educator in England, conducted comparative research and published and lectured internationally on childbearing and the ways in which women in different cultures feel about their bodies (Kitzinger, 1967). Others in the network of researchers, practitioners, and activists committed to improving maternity care included Dr. Pierre Vellay in France, Dr. Roberto Caldyro-Barcia in Latin America, Drs. Niles and Michael Newton, Ruth Lubic, Dr. John Seldon Miller, Flora Hommel, and Norma Swenson (Sakala & Swenson, 1999). Many others, professionals as well as parents, too numerous to mention made significant contributions to humanizing maternity care through their research, writings, speeches, and activism.

At the same time that professionals were speaking out for family-centered maternity care, the consumer movement continued with growth in membership and influence of ICEA, ASPO, and AAHCC. Many hospitals altered their physical surroundings and revised their policies and procedures in response to these influences and thus appeared to be more consumer friendly. Father participation in the role of labor coach became commonplace in the late 1970s. Visitation policies began to include siblings and other family members in the postpartum period (Wertz & Wertz, 1989). Rooming-in with the newborn was permitted in many hospitals, and attempts were made to accommodate consumer requests (Wertz & Wertz, 1989).

Alternative Birth Centers or Rooms

One outgrowth of the consumer, natural childbirth, and feminist movements of the 1960s was a resurgence of midwife-attended home birth. This development alarmed doctors who believed that birth outside of a hospital was unacceptably risky. Some hospitals responded to families' desire for a less institutional experience by opening alternative birth centers (ABCs), also called "birth rooms." ABCs offered homelike environments in hospitals, usually on the maternity unit. Certain families could be admitted to the ABC room, labor and give birth there, and then be sent home from it.

Families interested in this alternative to conventional hospital birth had to meet special hospital criteria, which usually included attendance in childbirth preparation classes, desire for non-medicated labor and birth, family participation, and being categorized in a medically low-risk designation (Phillips, 1996). Since obstetric interventions (other than episiotomy) were typically not permitted, deviations from normal labor resulted in immediate transfer of the woman to a conventional maternity unit. In part because of these restrictions and requirements, few physicians encouraged their patients to use ABCs, few families desired this option, and fewer still qualified. In many hospitals, these birth rooms were seldom used.

Development of LDR Rooms

By the 1980s, more than a third of the nation's hospitals had a designated "birthing center" or ABC (*American Journal of Public Health,* 1987). As ABCs grew in number, clinical experience proved these settings to be safe and satisfactory for both healthcare providers and families. The lessons learned from these units, as well as from other models of care from abroad, were incorporated into clinical practice and new facility designs.

Dr. Morris Notelovitz introduced the concept of the combination labor/delivery/recovery (LDR) room in 1970 at Addington Hospital in Durban, South Africa (Notelovitz, 1978). This "single unit delivery system" (SUDS) was designed for both low- and high-risk mothers to labor, deliver, and recover in one room before moving to another room for postpartum care. In the LDR system, the three separate multitransfer divisions are retained. After birth in an LDR room, the mother is moved to a postpartum room in a separate unit staffed by a separate nursing staff. In addition, the newborn is moved to a separate well-baby nursery staffed by yet another group of nurses.

Meanwhile in April 1969, under the guidance of Dr. Phillip Sumner, Manchester Memorial Hospital in Connecticut established homelike labor and delivery rooms where all women, low or high risk, could both labor and give birth. In 1976, Sumner reported on 6 years of successful obstetric practice in these LDR rooms (Sumner, 1976).

In August 1980, a Ross Planning Associates publication, *Alternatives for Obstetric Design*, described the LDR room (Basler, Hager, & Tienprasid, 1980). The authors utilized Notelovitz's concept, which combines labor, delivery, and recovery functions into one room.

Single-Room Maternity Care

In 1974, Fenwick developed the "Single-Room Maternity Care" (SRMC) concept, and in 1979 he authored an article entitled "Blueprint for the Humanization of American Obstetric Practice" (NAPSAC, 1979). By that time, the major maternal and infant professional organizations in the United States had published the joint statement on family-centered maternity care (1978), and American families had begun their effort to put the family back into the birth experience. Fenwick's article acknowledged this societal revolution and went beyond the limited response of ABCs and LDRs. He described a new system of care that included the benefits of family-centered maternity care as well as combined labor, delivery, recovery, and postpartum care in clusters of labor/delivery/recovery/postpartum (LDRP) rooms.

It is not uncommon to hear systems described as "LDRs" or "LDRPs." This terminology identifies a type of room as the key to the difference between a modified multitransfer system with LDRs and an SRMC program, and reflects confusion between a facility layout and a system of care (Box 1-2).

To facilitate implementation of his concept, Fenwick subsequently designed the first birthing bed that allowed the mother to change positions for labor and birth. In 1980, he published an article on the SRMC "cluster" concept for birth (Borning, 1980).

At this point, there was professional and consumer agreement that something had to be done to improve the American maternity care system, particularly the hospital birth environment. Although various alternatives—including the ABCs, Notelovitz's SUDS, and Fenwick's SRMC—had been introduced, there was no forum for professionals who were interested in

BOX 1-2

LDRs and LDRPs

An LDR room is a *component* of a multitransfer *system* that moves the family for care, which is provided by two or three nursing staff divisions.

An LDRP room is a *component* of the SRMC *system* in which multiskilled nurses provide care to the woman without moving her.

When a hospital identifies its maternity service as "LDRPs," it is a good indicator that the maternity service may not have fully grasped the programmatic characteristics of SRMC and may be experiencing difficulties in its implementation.

these new approaches to maternity care. There was also little, if any, research to support a change from the conventional maternity model or available assistance to develop or implement new ideas.

The Role of the Cybele Society

In the fall of 1979, the Cybele Society was founded to research and promote family-centered maternity care. This organization was established as a forum for a wide representation of maternity care providers, including obstetricians, pediatricians, nurses, midwives, anesthesiologists, family practitioners, and hospital administrators.

The Cybele Society's goal was to make Family-Centered Maternity Care (FCMC) standard practice, not the alternative that it was perceived to be at the time. The society was dedicated to the research and promotion of enlightened, rehumanized, and safe maternity care. Cybele's leadership understood that, in addition to a philosophy of FCMC, healthcare providers needed practical knowledge, skills, and tools that would enable them to develop workable strategies within their organizations and professional worlds. The Cybele Society provided education and a forum for the development of tools and served as a repository for information on SRMC from a variety of research and professional sources.

In 1981, the Cybele Society published a monograph titled *The Cybele Cluster: A Single-Room Maternity Care System for High- and Low-Risk Families.* Patient care rooms were clustered around a central service and nursing core area. These LDRP rooms were designed for nontransfer of the mother and baby during the entire maternity stay (Fenwick & Dearing, 1981).

The Cybele Society became both a platform and a catalyst for change by drawing together resources to allow the development of physical capabilities that would support the proposed changes in care delivery. The society's work came to the attention of the Kaiser Family Foundation, which sponsored a forum of nationally respected healthcare providers representing obstetrics, pediatrics, anesthesiology, hospital administration, maternity nursing, and medical ethics. This team conducted a formal review of all the possible approaches to maternity care and concluded that SRMC represented the best model for American maternity care in the future.

The National Perinatal Demonstration Project

Based on the Kaiser Family Foundation's endorsement, the Cybele Society set out to develop the National Perinatal Demonstration Unit to research the possible benefits of the SRMC program. This demonstration unit was to be established with a community hospital, utilizing a research protocol to obtain scientifically valid information about SRMC. The project's goals included improving the quality of childbirth care, reducing the cost of services, and increasing patient satisfaction with maternity care (Cybele Society, 1980). Unfortunately, due to a series of circumstances, including change of hospital ownership, the demonstration unit never became a reality. Consequently, there has not been an opportunity to validate the benefits of SRMC in a controlled demonstration project.

The First SRMC Programs

The Birthplace at St. Mary's Hospital in Minneapolis, Minnesota, and the St. Frances Regional

Medical Center in Shakopee, Minnesota, took the lead and implemented the first SRMC services. Both realized significant staff savings over the conventional obstetric system. By 1987, St. Mary's Hospital had also experienced a 41 percent increase in census (Phillips, 1988).

OUR BUSINESS: FAMILY BEGINNINGS

As described earlier, numerous maternity care professional organizations have long called for the provision of family-centered care. Indeed, *Guidelines for Perinatal Care* (1997)—developed through the cooperative efforts of the American Academy of Pediatrics (AAP) Committee on Fetuses and Newborns and the American College of Obstetricians and Gynecologists (ACOG) Committee on Obstetric Practice—recommends that the healthcare system be oriented toward providing family-centered care and emphasizes the social and psychological needs of mothers, infants, and families in childbirth in addition to appropriate medical care (Young, 1988). The Coalition for Improving Maternity Services (CIMS) has declared its mission to promote a wellness model of maternity care that will improve birth outcomes and substantially reduce costs. The coalition is composed of individuals and national organizations with a concern for the care and well-being of mothers, babies, and families (The Mother-Friendly Childbirth Initiative, 1996).

The World Health Organization (WHO) published an important report, *Care in Normal Birth: A Practical Guide,* in Geneva in 1996. The report addresses issues of care in normal birth irrespective of the birth setting or level of care. The aim of care in normal birth is "to achieve a healthy mother and child with the least possible level of intervention that is compatible with safety" (WHO, 1996). Also, the American College of Nurse-Midwives (ACNM), the American Nurses Association (ANA), and the Association of Women's Health, Obstetric and Neonatal Nurses (AWHONN) have long supported family-centered maternity care.

Maternity care professionals are in an optimum position to facilitate the development of stronger, more knowledgeable, and competent families through the provision of family-centered care throughout the childbearing year.

SAFETY AND SATISFACTION

Family-centered maternity care offers many benefits for families. A growing body of research indicates that family-centered care is cost-effective, is associated with better patient outcomes, and produces greater patient and provider satisfaction (Enkin, Keirse, Renfrew, & Neilson, 1995; Tomlinson et al., 1996; Institute for Family-Centered Care, 1998).

Implementing contemporary maternity services has long been challenged on the grounds that they are not proven to be safe. This concern is not valid. Articles concerning medical safety, staff and patient satisfaction of LDRs and medical safety, staff and patient satisfaction, and cost efficiency of SRMC began appearing in the literature in the 1980s and 1990s (Schmidt, 1983; Nathanson, 1985; *OB.GYN News*, 1985; Waryas & Luebbers, 1986; Reed & Schmid, 1986; Bajo, 1986; Bajo & Phillips, 1986; Beaver & Boehm, 1986; Phillips, 1986; Jones, 1987; Mitchell, 1987; Super, 1987; Phillips, 1988; Perry, 1989; Machol, 1989; *NAAWHP* Focus, 1990; Perry, 1990; Coile, 1990; Gardner, 1990; Williams & Mervis, 1990; Bishop, 1991; Yates & Mertel, 1991; Olson & Smith, 1992). All reported that there had been no increases in maternal or infant infection rates as strict gowning, draping and visitation policies were liberalized, and none found any detriment to maternal and newborn outcomes.

SUMMARY

At the beginning of the 20th century, women gave birth in their own homes in a familiar environment surrounded and supported by family and friends. However, if a serious problem occurred, little could be done. Hospitalization brought new remedies for pain, a means of monitoring the mother and child's well-being, treatments for complications, and reduction in maternal and infant mortality. Unfortunately, with safer birth through hospitalization came the medicalization of normal childbirth, a bureaucratic institutional structure, depersonalization, and fragmentation of care. The result was an unnecessary loss of social support that is so important to people as they make the transition to parenthood.

By the end of the 1970s, the major professional organizations involved in providing maternity and newborn care had called for a family-centered approach to maternity care. The SRMC program and facility design was introduced and was evaluated as being the best model for providing safe, satisfying, and cost-effective maternity care. As the 21st century begins, numerous maternity care organizations and individuals are again calling for the provision of family-centered maternity care. If we believe that birth is foremost a family's beginning, then it follows that we are in the business of family beginnings. In SRMC we have a method and a means to achieve this mission.

REFERENCES

American Academy of Pediatrics and American College of Obstetricians and Gynecologists (1997). *Guidelines for perinatal care* (4th ed.). Elk Grove, IL: American Academy of Pediatrics.

Bajo, K. (1986). Single-room maternity care. *Frontline, 4,* 2–5.

Bajo, K., & Phillips, C.R. (1986). Changing times and changing opportunities: Innovative maternity facility designs and the childbirth educator. *NAACOG Update Series* (Vol. 5, lesson 18). Princeton: Continuing Professional Education Center, Inc.

Basler, D.S., Hager, D.E., & Tienprasid, B. (1980). *Alternatives for obstetric design.* Columbus, OH: Ross Laboratories.

Beaver, V.S. & Boehm, F.H. (1986). Birth rooms in a teaching hospital: Initial 18 months' experience. *Perinatology-Neonatology,* 25–27.

Bishop, J.L. (1991). Single-room maternity can add flexibility. *Modern Healthcare's Facilities Operation and Management,* 12–14.

Borning Corporation (1980). *Nurture, 1*(4).

Bradley, R. (1981). *Husband-coached childbirth* (3rd ed.). New York: Harper and Row.

Coile, R.C., Jr. (1990). Obstetrics: Strategic centerpiece of "full service" hospitals in the 1990s. *Hospital Strategy Report, 2*(12), 3–8.

Colman, A., & Colman, L. (1971). *Pregnancy: The psychological experience*. New York: Seabury Press.

Cybele Society (1980). Unpublished material describing a national demonstration unit. Spokane, WA: Author.

De Lee, J.B. (1927). How should the maternity be isolated? *Modern Hospital, 29*(3), 65–72.

De Lee, J.B. (1927). *Obstetrics for Nurse-Obstetric Operations* (8th ed.). Philadelphia: W.B. Saunders.

De Lee, J.B. (1927). What are the special needs of modern maternity? *Modern Hospital, 27*(8), 59–69.

Dick-Read, G. (1953). *Childbirth without fear*. New York: Harper and Row.

Enkin, M., Keirse, M.J.N.C., Renfrew, M.J., & Neilson, J.A. (1995). *A guide to effective care in pregnancy and childbirth* (2nd ed.). New York: Oxford University Press.

Ewy, D., & Youmans, J.M. (1988). The early parenting experience. In F.H. Nichols & S.S. Humenick (Eds.), *Childbirth education: Practice, research and theory*. Philadelphia: W.B. Saunders.

Fenwick, L. (1979). Blueprint for the humanization of American obstetric practice. In D. Stewart & L. Stewart (Eds.), *Compulsory hospitalization: Freedom of choice in childbirth*. Marble Hill, MO: NAPSAC.

Fenwick, L., & Dearing, R.H. (1981). *The Cybele Cluster: A single room maternity care system for high- and low-risk families*. Spokane, WA: The Cybele Society.

Fenwick, L., & Simkin, P. (1987). Maternal positioning to prevent or alleviate dystocia in labor. *Clinical Obstetrics and Gynecology, 30*(1), 83–89.

Gardner, E. (1990). There's one more place like home. *Modern Healthcare's Facilities Operation and Management*, 24–27.

Haire, D., & Haire, J. (1968). *Implementing family-centered maternity care with a central nursery*. Bellevue, WA: ICEA.

Interprofessional Task Force on Health Care of Women and Children (1978). *A joint position statement on the development of family-centered maternity/newborn care in hospitals*. Chicago: American College of Obstetricians and Gynecologists.

Jones, C. (1987). Developing a successful alternative maternity unit. *Health Care Strategic Management*, 19–21.

Kay, M.A. (1982). *Anthropology of human birth*. Philadelphia: F.A. Davis.

Kitzinger, S. (1967). *The experience of childbirth*. Baltimore: Penguin Books.

Klaus, M.H., & Kennell, J.H. (1982). *Parent–infant bonding* (2nd ed.). St. Louis: C.V. Mosby.

Leavitt, J.W. (1989). Joseph B. DeLee and the practice of preventative obstetrics. *Obstetrical and Gynecological Survey, 44*(9), 682–683.

Machol, L. (1989). Single-room maternity care gains converts. *Contemporary Ob/Gyn, 29*, 62–64, 67, 70.

May, K. (1982). Three phases in the development of father involvement in pregnancy. *Nursing Research, 31*(6), 377–379.

Mitchell, C.F. (1987). Many hospitals replace traditional mode of maternity care with one-room plan. *Wall Street Journal*, November 27, p. 13.

Mother-Friendly Childbirth Initiative (1996). *The Coalition for Improving Maternity Services (CIMS)*. Washington, DC: Author.

Nathanson, M. (1985). Single-room maternity care seen as way to attract patients, cut costs. *Modern Healthcare, 15*(7), 72, 74.

Nichols, F.H., & Humenick, S.S. (1988). *Childbirth education: Practice, research, and theory*. Philadelphia: W.B. Saunders.

Notelovitz, M. (1978). The single-unit delivery system—a safe alternative to home deliveries. *American Journal of Obstetrics and Gynecology, 132*, 889–894.

Obstetrics department has become a big marketing tool of hospitals. (1985). *Ob. Gyn. News, 20*(14), 1, 20.

Olson, M.E., & Smith, M.J. (1992). An evaluation of single-room maternity care. *Health Care Supervisor, 11*(1), 43–49.

Parturition: Places and priorities [editorial]. (1987). *American Journal of Public Health, 77*(8), 923.

Perry, L. (1989). Nurturing single-room maternity care. *Modern Healthcare, 19*(19), 18–19, 22, 24–25.

Perry, L. (1990). Single-room maternity care begets more utilization. *Modern Healthcare, 20*(5), 46.

Perry, L. (1990). Single-room maternity plan pleases nurses. *Modern Healthcare, 20*(20), 44.

Perry, P. (1990). Market memo: The obstetrics market matures for LDRs/LDRPs. *Health Care Strategic Management, 8*(4), 1, 19–22.

Phillips, C.R. (1986). Problems and solutions in innovative maternity programs. *Frontline, 4*, 6–8.

Phillips, C.R. (1988). Single-room maternity care for maximum cost-efficiency. *Perinatology-Neonatology*, March/April.

Phillips, C.R. (1996). *Family-centered maternity and newborn care: A basic text* (4th ed.). St. Louis: C.V. Mosby.

Phillips, C.R., & Anzalone, J.T. (1978). *Fathering: Participation in labor and birth*. St. Louis: C.V. Mosby.

Phillips, C.R., & Anzalone, J. (1982). *Fathering: Participation in labor and birth* (2nd ed.). St. Louis: C.V. Mosby.

Porges, R.F. (1985). The response of the New York Obstetrical Society to the report by the New York Academy of Medicine on maternal mortality, 1933–1934. *American Journal of Obstetrics and Gynecology, 152*(6), 642–649.

Reed, G., & Schmid, M. (1986). Nursing implementaion of single-room maternity care. *Journal of Obstetric, Gynecologic, and Neonatal Nursing, 15*, 386–389.

Rooks, J.P. (1997). *Midwifery and childbirth in America*. Philadelphia: Temple University Press.

Rubin, R. (1970). Cognitive style in pregnancy. *American Journal of Nursing, 70*, 502.

Rubin, R. (1975). Maternal tasks in pregnancy. *Maternal-Child Nursing Journal, 4*(3), 143–153.

Sakala, C., & Swenson, N. (1999). Murray Enkin. Celebration and tribute. *Birth, 26*(1), 1–3.

Schmidt, R.T.F. (1983). Labor-delivery-recovery room: Planning the delivery suite for current need. *Clinics in Perinatology, 10*(1), 49–59.

Shultz, D.G. (1958). Cruelty in the maternity wards. *Ladies Home Journal*, May, 44–45, 152–155.

Single-room maternity care brings more patients and higher staff satisfaction (1990). *NAWHP Focus, 7*.

Speert, H. (1980). *Obstetrics and gynecology in America—a history*. Chicago: American College of Obstetricians and Gynecologists.

Sumner, P.E. (1976). Six years experience of prepared childbirth in a home-like labor-delivery room. *Birth and the Family Journal, 3*(2), 79–82.

Super, K.E. (1987). Single-room maternity care aiding hospitals. *Modern Healthcare, 17*(46), 128.

Tomlinson, P.S., Mattson Bryan, A.A., & Lash Esau, A. (1996). Family-centered intrapartum care: Revisiting an old concept. *Journal of Obstetric, Gynecologic, and Neonatal Nursing, 25*(4), 331–337.

Waryas, F.S., & Luebbers, F.S. (1986). A cluster system for maternity care. *American Journal of Maternal/Child Nursing, 11*(2), 98–100.

Wertz, R.W., & Wertz, D.C. (1989). *Lying-in: A history of childbirth in America* (expanded edition). New Haven: Yale University Press.

What the Research Shows. In *Advances in family-centered care*,(4),1. Bethesda, MD: Institute for Family-Centered Care.

Wiedenbach, E. (1959). *Family-centered maternity nursing*. New York: G.P. Putnam.

Williams, J.K., & Mervis, M.R. (1990). Use of the labor-delivery-recovery room in an urban tertiary care hospital. *American Journal of Obstetrics and Gynecology, 162*, 23–24.

World Health Organization (1966). *Care in normal birth: A practical guide*. Report of a Technical Working Group. Publication no. WHO/FRH/MSM/96.24. Geneva: WHO.

Yates, M.J., & Mertel, W.G. (1991). LDRP: That's the acronym for giving birth in style. *Puget Sound Business Journal*, March 25, p. 21.

Young, D. (1998). [Review of the book *Guidelines for perinatal care*]. *Birth, 25*(2), 135–137.

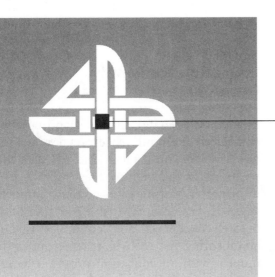

CHAPTER 2

The SRMC Program

WHAT DOES "SRMC" MEAN?

Throughout this book, the acronym SRMC stands for Single-Room Maternity Care. As explained previously, SRMC is a comprehensive, socially responsive maternity care program that is provided in a nontransfer facility designed to optimize family beginnings.

SRMC incorporates and operationalizes the philosophical foundation of family-centered maternity care. SRMC has defined goals, principles, and practices to support the family's physical, psychological, and developmental needs during the childbearing year. SRMC defines a continuum of care that begins before conception, includes early prenatal care, and proceeds through the childbearing year. This requires a level and scope of practice that goes beyond conventional medical and nursing care.

We use the acronym SRMC when referring to a defined program of maternity care provided in a nontransfer facility model. When discussing the physical facility or program alone, we refer to it either as the SRMC facility or the SRMC program.

SRMC PROGRAM GOALS

SRMC provides a comprehensive program of physical, psychological, and developmental support during the childbearing year. The goal is

healthy mothers and healthy babies; parents who can successfully parent their babies through the first year; parents who make conception, pregnancy, birth, and childcare choices that are in the best interests of the baby and family; and families that are nurturing and enduring.

SRMC COMPONENTS

Single-room maternity care is characterized by a comprehensive approach to fostering optimal family beginnings during the childbearing year and by a program and facility that keep the family together, in a single room, throughout the hospital portion of their maternity care. The main components of SRMC include culturally sensitive inclusion of the family, education for family development, and multidisciplinary normalcy-oriented maternity and newborn care.

Inclusion of Family

Promoting full family participation during childbirth can foster family stability and a better environment for children (Tomlinson, 1996). The family is the oldest human institution. It is society's most basic unit, surviving throughout the centuries because it serves vital human needs. Although there may be different styles of family living and different ways of relating the family to the society, the family will continue to exist in some form as long as the human race exists on earth (Mead, 1965).

Family can be defined legally, morally, socially, psychologically, and functionally (Kuhn, 1984). It is impossible to describe a "typical" family today. Family types may include nuclear families, extended families, single-parent families, and blended families. For purposes of this book, a family is defined as those persons who are identified by the childbearing woman as providing familial support, whether or not they are biologically related.

Although only the woman is physically pregnant, family members also experience shifts and changes in feelings, relationships, and lifestyle associated with pregnancy and a child's impending birth. An SRMC program includes the people who live with the mother and love her. Excluding these people deprives the mother of her most important support system and fragments her care.

Meeting the Needs of Different Cultures

The trend for the 21st century will be toward greater ethnic, cultural, and religious diversity, with people maintaining their cultural identities while participating in American life. Because SRMC programs offer individualized care, healthcare professionals who provide it can be sensitive and responsive to the beliefs, values, and customs that are specific to each mother's culture, ethnic group, and/or religion. SRMC programs prepare clinical staff members (physicians, nurses, and support staff) to care for this increasingly diverse population by educating staff about varied health beliefs, practices, and mores of specific ethnic and cultural groups. Staff members are also given the opportunity to look at ways their own cultures affect their views of what is important. Such a perspective helps healthcare professionals see that each patient embodies a unique cultural heritage. Because SRMC does not require families to transfer from the care of the nurses who have cared for them during labor and birth, it fosters trust and rapport and facilitates understanding various families' cultural mores.

Education for Family Development

Pregnancy, prenatal, birthing, and newborn care choices strongly influence pregnancy and family development outcomes. The SRMC education program is tailored to meet family needs for information during each of these important life stages. It is a comprehensive program that begins before conception and continues through the childbearing year. SRMC reaches out to the community with an education program to influence family choices. Although the choice of when to start a family may be difficult to influence in some places, the maternity program's potential influence becomes strong once parents-to-be seek prenatal care. Behavioral and maternity care choices made during this stage can have an important effect on future care options and results.

Nontransfer

Not having to move the family from room to room and from nurse to nurse facilitates communication, continuity of care, and education during the hospital stay. It also facilitates safety, cost efficiency, and staff satisfaction as well as reducing labor, space, and equipment requirements.

Enhanced Efficiency of Space and Staffing

By consolidating the separate labor, delivery, recovery, and postpartum phases, SRMC reduces total space requirements as well as the number of full-time equivalents (FTEs) necessary to provide full family care (Figure 2-1).

Normalcy-Oriented Maternity and Newborn Clinical Care

A normalcy-oriented maternity and newborn care program, based on evidence-based, physiologic management, is key to making childbirth safer and more comfortable, controlling unnecessary procedures and costs, and developing the family's self-confidence (Simpson & Knox,

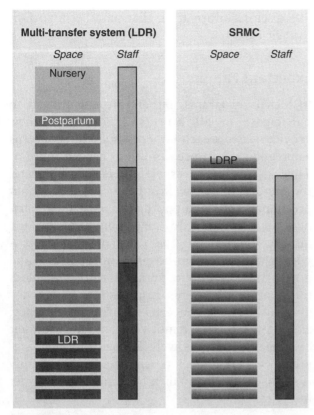

FIGURE 2–1. Comparison of multi-transfer system (LDR) with SRMC system.

1999). A normalcy-based program also facilitates education by fostering a more comfortable recovery. SRMC emphasizes physiologic management of labor and birth and thus reduces the need for intervention.

Multidisciplinary Care

The SRMC clinical team is responsive to the woman and her family. According to the setting, the team may include obstetricians, pediatricians, family physicians, anesthesiologists, certified registered nurse anesthetists (CRNAs), certified nurse-midwives (CNMs), nurse-practitioners (NPs), registered nurses (RNs), nutritionists, social workers, childbirth educators, case managers, and community or outreach workers, who all share SRMC's goals. Women and their families can serve as advisors to the SRMC team to help evaluate the effectiveness of program changes.

THE SRMC PROGRAM

Healthy pregnancies begin well in advance of conception. Ideally, an SRMC program begins before conception and extends through the childbearing year.

Preconception Care

The goal of preconception care is to ensure that a woman is healthy and knowledgeable prior to pregnancy and to identify risk factors related to poor pregnancy outcome (Frede & Strohbach, 1992). The SRMC program endeavors to establish healthcare protocols that are in the best interest of the woman and her family and to promote empowerment for women and their partners as they make reproductive choices and decisions. Completion of a preconception medical and psychosocial risk assessment permits the discovery and treatment of underlying health problems. Thus, interventions can be designed to reduce psychosocial risks and promote general health and well-being. All of these can improve pregnancy outcomes (Frede & Strohbach, 1992).

Preconception care includes preconception education and counseling services. These offerings focus on promotion of healthful behaviors, provide general knowledge of pregnancy and parenting, and impart information on personal care and community resources. Content is presented regarding family planning, infertility problems, and genetic counseling. When this is inconsistent with the organizations' values, families are directed to sources of information should they ask for it.

Women and their partners can receive assistance in selecting a physician or midwife and a facility at which to give birth. Preconception education has an added marketing value because couples are likely to come to the sponsoring hospital for care once they are pregnant.

Information about breastfeeding can be presented during preconception education and care. Most parents decide whether to breastfeed by early pregnancy, often before the first prenatal visit or class. Prenatal intent is a strong predictor of breastfeeding outcome (Canadian Institute of

Child Health, 1996). Therefore, educators and healthcare providers should explore breastfeeding attitudes and knowledge with potential parents. The preconception period is, perhaps, an ideal time to correct myths and give couples information that will help them make an informed decision about breastfeeding.

Whether a woman has a healthy pregnancy depends largely on her success in taking good care of herself. This includes proper exercise, nutrition, and other preventive measures such as avoiding sources of infections like toxoplasmosis or listeria. It may include smoking cessation, reduction in stress, and elimination of substance and alcohol abuse. All of these factors not only improve health but also can substantially reduce costs of maternity care.

Antepartum Care

The goal of antepartum care in any setting is to improve and maintain the health and well-being of the mother, her unborn child, and her family. To do this, most programs address the emotional, psychosocial, biological, and medical aspects of pregnancy, childbirth, and parenting for pregnant women and their families. SRMC programs further emphasize the goal of empowering women and their families to make informed decisions about all aspects of care during the childbearing year. To accomplish this goal, providers practicing in SRMC programs collaborate to provide high-quality, evidence-based clinical care and integrate specific educational content designed to inform expectant mothers and their families about the unique events of the childbearing year.

SRMC antepartum care programs use the process of risk screening to further the education of women and their families and to help them plan for their needs throughout pregnancy and after childbirth. Because SRMC programs emphasize early infant developmental needs, home health providers—as well as medical staff providers—continue this emphasis on education and empowerment for the childbearing year. In SRMC programs, providers make every effort to establish an atmosphere of mutual trust and respect between families and care providers. This helps to create an atmosphere in which women can disclose information that may be important to their care.

Expectant Fathers

In SRMC programs, fathers are encouraged to participate in all aspects of the pregnancy. Providers assess each father's issues and concerns as pregnancy advances and offer needed support. They also help expectant fathers to understand the importance of healthy behaviors throughout pregnancy and to support and assist their partners in self-care. To help communicate the father's concerns to the team of professionals who will provide in-hospital intrapartum and postpartum care, the prenatal record includes information about his responses to pregnancy and his stated concerns. During pregnancy, expectant fathers are motivated to improve their own health status as well. Recognizing their significance to the development of a healthy family is sufficient for many men to commit to healthier lifestyles.

Family Attachment

Attachment is the process of forming an enduring bond between parents and babies (Todd, 1998). Examples follow that demonstrate how caregivers can facilitate attachment during the antenatal period. The father is encouraged to attend the first antepartum visit. He is included as an integral part of the care process and encouraged to show continued interest. Care providers can encourage other family members to accompany the woman on antepartum visits. Children in the family can assist with care procedures, feel fetal movements, listen to the fetal heartbeat, and learn about pregnancy and the birth process, all of which can help them form a bond with their unborn sibling. It may be necessary to schedule appointments on weekend days and evenings to provide times when family members can be present, but the benefits to the family are well worth the inconvenience to providers.

Care providers can also educate families about fetal growth and development. Most families will be fascinated to know that from the sixth month of pregnancy (and perhaps earlier), the fetus is capable of seeing, hearing, tasting, and responding (Goer, 1989). Families can be encouraged to talk and sing to the baby and to play with the baby by patting or gently palpating the mother's belly.

Informed Decision Making

A basic tenet of family-centered antepartum care is that decisions about care should be made collaboratively. Some families prefer to leave all decisions up to their doctor or midwife; however, most welcome and appreciate the opportunity to explore the pros and cons of their various options under a trusted medical professional's guidance. Although this can be time consuming, good, open communication between care provider and family is the best way to develop a trusting relationship. The antepartum period offers many opportunities for providers to give parents the information they need to learn about the influence of the new family member on their lives.

This is the time for providers to educate couples about normal pregnancy, labor, birth, and parenting. Emphasis is on pregnancy not as a disease state but as a state of wellness, during which individuals move from the role of expectant parents to the role and responsibilities of parents of a new baby.

Preparation for labor and birth goes beyond education about relaxation, breathing, and pushing techniques to discussion of the benefits and risks of various medical interventions, including analgesia and anesthesia for labor and birth. It is important for SRMC programs to provide education about physiologic labor support techniques, the importance of ambulation and position changes in labor, and the use of the birthing bed as a labor support tool (Figure 2-2). Parents need information about bonding, attachment, and the importance of extensive, close physical contact between mother and baby so that they understand the new relationship and are prepared to keep the infant with them at all times following birth. This will also help prepare parents for the practice of mother–baby care so that they appreciate the value of having the baby at the mother's bedside instead of in the nursery.

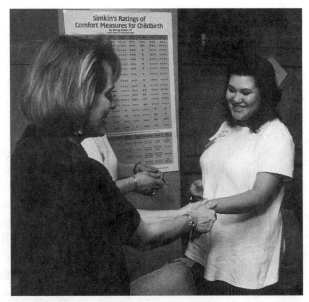

FIGURE 2–2. Birth class provides education about physiologic labor support techniques. (Photo courtesy of the Family Maternity Center, Evergreen Hospital Medical Center, Kirkland, WA.)

Because education is such an important aspect of antepartum care, all members of the clinical staff, including physicians, nurses, and support staff, must be knowledgeable about and support the philosophy of the SRMC program. They must understand and be prepared to present factual, objective information at every interaction with the childbearing family.

Birth Plans

In addition to engaging in dialogue about diagnostic and treatment options for the intrapartum and postpartum periods, providers also invite discussion of the woman's attitudes, fears, preferences, and desires about the birth experience. This process allows providers to present the pros and cons of medical and nursing procedures as they relate to maternal–infant bonding and attachment, family formation, and attaining parenting skills. Armed with this information, parents can put their preferences into a written birth plan and give that plan to the hospital staff so that all providers who come in contact with the family will know their preferences. The birth plan is a tangible tool that allows women to actively participate in decisions regarding their care. It also provides an opportunity for families to discuss and negotiate care practices with practitioners *before* the woman arrives in labor (Carty & Tier, 1989). Birth plans are especially important when the care provider who saw the woman during pregnancy may not attend her in labor.

A birth plan communicates "who I am, what is important to me, and why." The birth plan is written by the mother and family and contains their preferences, priorities, concerns, and goals for the birth and postpartum experience. It discusses preferences regarding pain medication and nonpharmacologic labor-coping techniques and the family's hopes regarding the working relationship with staff and caregivers. It should also include religious, cultural, and family traditions that the woman would like to or is obliged to observe during the birth experience (Phillips, 1994). Parents expecting a second or later baby may wish to include a brief description of previous experiences and their meaning in relation to the upcoming labor. The birth plan becomes a permanent part of the prenatal record and is sent from the provider's office to the birth facility along with the woman's history and physical forms.

Choosing Pediatric Care

During the pregnancy, families need to understand the importance of interviewing and selecting a pediatrician, family care physician, or nurse practitioner for newborn care. In almost all cases, data indicate that a mother's feeding decision is made early in pregnancy or, in many cases, before she becomes pregnant (Losch et al., 1995). Thus, the family and infant care provider should share similar philosophies regarding decision making, breastfeeding, and parenting in general.

Family Care Paths

The maternity care team, along with the family, develops a Family Care Path at the beginning of the antepartum period. This care path presents expected events, actions, and outcomes for mother and baby in a timeline representing the childbearing year. It defines the roles of team members and family members in order to enhance understanding of each individual's responsibilities and to help assure coordination of planned activities. All SRMC providers refer to and follow this care path throughout the childbearing year, and its use offers many opportunities for family education and participation in decision making about care.

Pre-admission Orientation

To help families prepare for the actual labor and birth and become more comfortable with the maternity care unit, SRMC programs invite small groups of expectant families to visit the childbirth facility. For their convenience, hospitals schedule tours at a variety of times, including evenings and weekends. The purpose of this tour is not to acquaint family members with policies, rules, and regulations, but to introduce families to staff members, to the system of care, and to resources. Further, family members become familiar with the facility, its physical layout, and features such as the patient/family resource library. A guide can explain the maternity program's components and provide information on the FCMC philosophy, present media materials, and explain consent procedures. The orientation tour also offers hospital staff and families an opportunity to discuss birth options and resources available both through the hospital and in the wider community. Families are given a copy of the hospital's maternity care philosophy. This is also the appropriate time for consultation with hospital business staff about financial arrangements, prepayment options, and insurance requirements.

Antepartum High-Risk Care

Some women may require prolonged hospitalization during pregnancy. To minimize stress, these women will need a quiet, nonthreatening environment in which close monitoring is possible. Women should receive individualized care so they can live their lives as normally and comfortably as possible given their medical condition. In SRMC programs, family visiting and participation in care are encouraged. Space is provided so that each woman's partner and/or family members can remain overnight.

When possible, SRMC programs design and implement antepartum home care programs for women with high-risk pregnancies. Whether in-hospital or home-based, care plans address issues arising from the disruption of the family's lives and their emotional distress. Referrals to community services and social services are also important.

Intrapartum Care

The goal of intrapartum care in SRMC programs is to provide a safe and satisfying birth that supports the normalcy of the birth experience and empowers the family. SRMC intrapartum care emphasizes the inclusion of fathers or other family members and friends in the process to the extent that they and the mother desire (Figure 2-3). This may include children. Family-centered care during labor and birth offers many options to the childbearing family. Even when medical intervention is required, providers take care to preserve as many of these options as possible.

High-Risk Intrapartum Care

Women at high risk need family-centered care as much as or more than women with normal preg-

nancies because they face additional psychological challenges. High-tech care does not preclude high-touch care. Staff members are educated to give culturally competent care. In regions where large numbers of patients have limited English skills, the hospital trains staff members in the rudiments of the main languages spoken locally and/or provides translators.

Empowerment

The mother's birth experience has profound and permanent effects on how she feels about the birth, herself, her partner, and her baby. The key component of a positive birth experience is a sense of mastery and a feeling that she coped well and was an active participant in decisions (Humenick & Bugen, 1981; Humenick, 1981; Simkin, 1991). Another essential component is that she is nurtured and supported by those caring for her (Simkin, 1991; Tarka & Paunonen, 1996; Hodnett, 1996; Bryanton, Fraser-Davey & Sullivan, 1994). The mother's and family's experiences of the birth, it should be added, also have long-term effects on their perceptions of the care they received (Fowles, 1998; Simkin, 1991; Simkin, 1992).

Hospital staff can help give the woman control over her experience in many ways. It can be something as small as asking a woman whether she wants to wear her own clothing or as signifi-

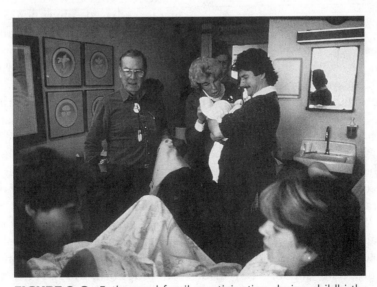

FIGURE 2–3. Father and family participation during childbirth.

cant as engaging the woman in resolving labor difficulties through position changes and activity. Barring emergencies, staff members pay meticulous attention to issues of informed decision making. In particular, they must understand and respect that refusal of various choices is valid.

Involvement of Support Person(s)

In SRMC programs, a woman is never routinely separated from her support person(s) at any time during labor or birth, including during a cesarean section. Staff members encourage the other parent or support person(s) to be present, as the mother desires and circumstances allow (AWHONN Standards and Guidelines, 1998).

Care Practices

SRMC programs stress the use of evidence to guide clinical practice; therefore, SRMC programs promote practices that support physiologic labor and birthing care along with normalcy-based maternal and newborn care. Care providers and nurses individualize care according to the SRMC program's goals and according to each woman's needs, wishes, and condition (AWHONN Standards and Guidelines, 1998). However, in the absence of research evidence, healthcare providers use their clinical judgment and experience to determine the "best practices" available.

Labor Support

In SRMC programs, physicians and nurses are educationally and experientially prepared to provide continuous emotional and physical support for laboring women. Studies have shown such support can reduce the need for pain medication, especially epidurals. Further, appropriate labor support can reduce the incidence of medical interventions, including cesarean birth, instrumental vaginal delivery, intravenous oxytocin, and episiotomy (Hodnett, 1999; Madi et al., 1999; Gordon et al., 1999; Gagnon, Waghorn, & Covell, 1997; Kennell & McGrath, 1993; Hodnett & Osborn, 1989). Appropriate support can also reduce the number of newborns who have low

APGAR scores, who require admission to special care nurseries, and who have longer than usual hospital stays (Hodnett, 1999; Kennell et al., 1991; Klaus et al., 1986; Cogan & Spinnato, 1988). In addition, women who receive continuous labor support experience less pain and anxiety in labor, feel a greater sense of control, and express greater satisfaction with the labor process. They are more likely to feel they coped well, have an easier time with mothering, and demonstrate better mothering skills. They also have higher self-esteem and experience less postpartum depression (Hodnett, 1999; Gordon et al., 1999; Martin et al., 1998). Obvious financial benefits for the hospital, as well as great psychosocial benefits for the woman and her family, result from shorter labors and fewer interventions.

Physiologic Labor and Birth Management

Abbie's birth (Figure 2-4) is an example of the experience that the SRMC program strives to provide. A woman, supported by her baby's father, experiences the personal triumph of giving birth while medical and nursing staff ensure, without intervening, that the experience is safe. The scientific rationale and clinical methods for assisting the normal processes of labor and birth are discussed in Chapter 3. A normalcy-oriented maternity and newborn care program, based on evidence-based, physiologic management, is key to making childbirth safer and more comfortable, controlling unnecessary procedures and costs, and developing the family's self-confidence. A normalcy-based program also makes resources available for education that supports family development by avoiding activities and costs that unnecessary procedures would have diverted.

Work-sampling studies show that even when a maternity unit is staffed with the goal of one-to-one nurse–patient ratios during active labor, nurses spend less than 10 percent of their time giving supportive care. Most of the time nurses spend with patients, in fact, falls into the category of providing "instruction/information" (Gagnon & Waghorn, 1996; McNiven, Hodnett, & O'Brien-Pallas, 1992). These findings are particu-

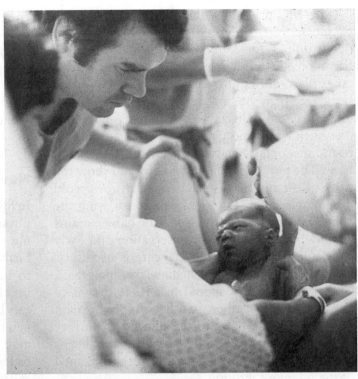

FIGURE 2–4. Abbie's Birth: A woman labors in the presence of her family and skilled assistants who support, encourage, and protect her. She responds to her body signals by walking, sitting, squatting, kneeling, or lying in various positions. In so doing, she directs the force of her contractions to angle and turn her baby through her pelvis. An assistant guides the infant's head, then shoulders, to prevent tearing during the woman's final, overwhelming urge to push. The mother reaches for her new baby and brings it to her face and breast. She has given birth and life. She is a mother. It is her personal triumph, a transforming moment that will be with her until the end of her days.

larly disturbing because of the benefits of supportive labor care, as noted above. Also, supporting women in labor may lead to a more cooperative and satisfying work environment for nurses (McNiven, Hodnett, & O'Brien-Pallas, 1992), as well as a more positive and satisfying birth experience for families.

It is possible to remedy some of this deficit. Educated in an era of "high-tech," low-touch care and nearly universal epidural use, many nurses and physicians lack basic labor support skills. However, they can be taught the importance of supportive care, and they can be educated to provide labor support techniques and nonpharmacologic pain management strategies. Educational programs can prepare them to implement strategies to promote labor progress.

Nonetheless, the heavy patient loads that are one result of staff reduction efforts may make one-to-one labor support impractical. A trained labor support specialist can fill this gap. Commonly known as a "doula" (from Greek, meaning "in service of"), these women provide physical and emotional support during labor and birth but do not assess the mother's or fetus's well-being (DONA, 1998). Generally, families engage the doula privately.

The "monitrice" (from French, meaning "to watch over attentively") is another labor-support professional. Generally a nurse or midwife, this individual combines nurturing skills with clinical assessment skills (Perez & Snedeker, 1990). The monitrice can provide actual care to the laboring woman. She can also assist and monitor women at home during early labor and help them determine when to come in to the hospital.

Cesarean Birth

In SRMC programs, cesarean births are a family-centered experience. Caregivers encourage the father or other support persons to be present during preparation for the surgery and during the cesarean birth. If possible, the cesarean birth takes place in an operating room located on the maternity unit instead of in general surgery. If the mother has no support person to accompany her through the surgical preparation and the operation, a staff member assumes the role of giving explanations and offering emotional support.

In SRMC programs, the clinical staff actively promotes early infant attachment by creating opportunities for families to interact from the first moments following birth. To ensure that this takes place during a cesarean birth, the anesthesia screen can be lowered at the time of the infant's actual delivery so the parents may view the birth. The mother's arms are freed from restraint so she can touch both the father and baby. The father may hold the baby and show the baby to the mother as she desires, or the screen may be placed so as to leave space for lying the baby across the mother's chest. The baby remains in the operating room for observation and early care unless immediate nursery care is necessary. Even a baby needing immediate transport to a special care nursery should briefly be shown to the mother. The father or other support person accompanies the baby to the nursery to further the attachment process. The clinical staff keeps the mother and other family members informed of the infant's condition.

It is particularly important that the father be present if the mother receives general anesthesia for a cesarean birth. This will give him the chance to participate in his child's birth and will provide him with the birth experience to share with the mother.

Following a cesarean birth, a mother receives all care during the immediate postoperative period in her labor-delivery-recovery-postpartum (LDRP) room if her condition and staffing levels permit. During this time, staff pays meticulous attention to post-surgical pain control, making every effort to keep the mother awake and aware so that she can participate in her infant's care, if only through observation. Injecting narcotic into the epidural catheter at the end of the surgery or supplying patient-controlled analgesia are two techniques that can keep mothers comfortable enough to care for their newborns and interact with their families. Cesarean mothers are encouraged to breastfeed and helped to find positions that avoid pressure on the incision during breastfeeding. Family members are encouraged to assist the mother in caring for the baby, remaining overnight if necessary to provide assistance to the mother so the baby can remain with her.

Women who have cesarean births often need extra emotional support. They may be grieving or disappointed, and these feelings should be accepted as healthy and normal. They will also need anticipatory guidance on coping with a newborn while recovering from major surgery and on what to expect physically and emotionally during the healing process (Goer, 1991).

Newborn Care

In SRMC programs, staff members promote close physical contact between mother and baby during the birth process and immediately following birth. The provider can guide the mother's hands to touch the infant being born. The mother can lift the baby, with the provider's assistance, and can lay the baby on her abdomen for immediate newborn care. The father or other support person may be invited to cut the cord after the physician or midwife has clamped it. Members of the clinical staff encourage both parents and other family members to touch and hold the infant during initial care procedures to encourage bonding and attachment.

Initial Newborn Care

The LDRP room's temperature is maintained at a level that prevents excessive cooling of the infant, and the baby is dried and placed skin-to-skin on the mother's or father's chest, with a warm cover over them. A dry stockinette cap on the baby's head retards heat loss, as do warmed blankets and a warming light placed over mother and baby.

Staff can care for the baby in the mother's or father's arms. Nurses can place identification tags, determine Apgar scores, and inject medications while one parent holds the baby. If the infant is at risk, unstable, or requires a greater degree of physical attention, nurses can place an infant warmer next to the mother's bed. This allows the baby to be next to the mother, at the side of her bed where she can see what is happening with her baby.

To promote eye contact between parents and their newborn at first meeting, the administration of ophthalmic eye ointment or eye drops can be delayed for at least 1 hour to allow unimpeded eye contact between parents and baby. Breast-feeding immediately after birth encourages lactation (American Academy of Pediatrics, 1997). In SRMC services, all nurses are educated in how to help new mothers get the baby started on the breast. In most cases, bathing the newborn is delayed until the body temperature normalizes approximately 2 to 6 hours following birth unless there is a medical indication to bathe the baby sooner.

In keeping with the emphasis on evidence-based practice, parents are informed of risks and benefits of circumcision. If parents opt for circumcision, use of a local anesthetic minimizes the infant's discomfort so there is little, if any, disruption in the attachment process (American Academy of Pediatrics, 1999).

Neonatal Intensive Care

Families of high-risk newborns lose the usual opportunity to hold, touch, and make eye contact with their babies—a problem that can interfere with the attachment process (Klaus, Kennell, & Klaus, 1995). These families also must struggle with their grief at losing the perfect child of their dreams and face the fear of losing the child to death. FCMC for high-risk newborns can help families with these issues.

Since the parents are responsible for providing lifelong physical and emotional care, all staff members treat the parents and their infants as a unit from the very beginning. Parents, siblings, and grandparents are encouraged to visit their baby in the neonatal intensive care nursery and to participate in the infant's care. It is important to encourage families to touch, hold, and care for their babies to the greatest extent possible. Loving touch and breastfeeding have psychosocial benefits and make an irreplaceable contribution to the infant's growth and health (Klaus, Kennell, & Klaus, 1995; Biancuzzo, 1999).

Special Care Nursery/ Neonatal Intensive Care Unit (NICU)

The advent of family-centered care has dramatically changed the special care of newborns toward a more baby- and family-friendly model in both facility design and clinical program. Historically, much of high-risk neonatal care's focus has been on medical intervention. Today, caregivers are beginning to recognize the importance of the nursery environment and the interactions of staff, families, and infants.

To implement family-centered care in high-risk nurseries, planners assess all aspects of care, including coordination of care. The goal is to create a supportive environment in which all neonates will have the best chance for optimal growth and development. Research has shown that developmental care practices in a family-centered environment lead to shorter hospital stays, fewer days on mechanical ventilation, faster weight gain, and fewer hospital readmissions in comparison with standard neonatal practices and environments (Grunwald & Becker, 1990).

A "supportive environment" includes human milk, especially the mother's own milk, as the food for any baby capable of oral intake. Human milk, especially the mother's own, is literally a life-saving therapy because of its anti-infective properties (Raisler & O'Campo, 1999). It also improves neurologic development. Any baby capable of sucking and swallowing is put to the breast. Breastfeeding causes less physiologic stress than bottle-feeding (Biancuzzo, 1995). SRMC programs encourage skin-to-skin or kangaroo pouching for infants capable of breathing room air; that is, the infant, dressed only in a diaper, is placed directly on top of the mother's bare chest and is then covered with the mother's clothing or a warmed blanket or both.

Parents must have information in words they can understand about the risks and benefits of various treatment options, including doing nothing. Refusal is a valid option. If they speak limited or no English, they must have information presented in their native language. All surgical procedures are done under proper anesthesia.

Postpartum Care

During the postpartum period, families go through major physiologic, psychological, and social adaptive processes. Successful mastery of this transition to parenthood creates the foundation for enduring, healthy family relationships

(Todd, 1998). The goal of family-centered post-partum care is to send parents home with beginning confidence in their ability to care for their infant and families who have begun the process of forming a strong attachment to the new baby.

In SRMC programs, families receive care as a unit. Nurses assist and encourage families to care for the woman and the baby. From the time of birth on, regardless of whether mother and baby are well, the mother, father, siblings, baby, and significant others are encouraged to remain together (Figure 2-5). Well babies are not admitted in a nursery; instead, they are formally admitted to the hospital in the mother's LDRP room. Every effort is made to equip the LDRP room so that a baby with special needs may be cared for at the mother's bedside. Only when complications cannot be taken care of in the mother's room, or equipment or staff are not available, will the baby be cared for in a special care nursery.

Whenever possible, staff provide all infant care at the mother's bedside, beginning during the immediate post-birth period. The maternity staff integrate education with care to prepare family members for the responsibilities of being parents, siblings, and grandparents of a new baby (Phillips, 1997). All clinical staff members acknowledge and treat babies as aware, sensitive human beings at the time of their births. To prepare mothers and fathers for their important roles as parents, discharge planning and referral services are essential to every SRMC program's success.

Visitors

Family members (as designated by the mother) are not considered visitors. They are free to come and go as the mother wishes. Partners are welcome to sleep in the LDRP room overnight. Family adaptation can be assisted by helping siblings to have a "birthday party" for the new baby and involving them in postpartum events, such as encouraging them to assist with infant footprinting or bathing.

Nonfamily members of the mother's choice are also welcome. Nursing staff members use their critical thinking and communication skills to help mothers determine when visitors are appropriate so that family–infant interaction is not disrupted.

Postpartum Education

Most parents have learned the basics of caring for their babies physically; however, they know little about what to expect from their newborn, what capabilities the newborn has, or how to read the

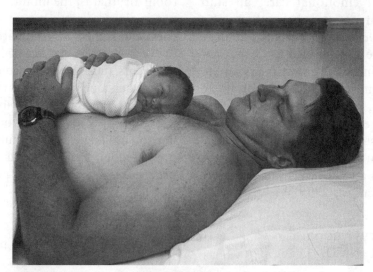

FIGURE 2–5. Father and baby. (Photo courtesy of the Family Maternity Center, Evergreen Hospital Medical Center, Kirkland, WA.)

baby's signals and effectively respond to his or her needs (Todd, 1998). For this reason, SRMC programs supplement traditional parent education about newborn bathing, temperature taking, umbilical cord care, and care of the intact or circumcised penis with education on newborn behavior, states of consciousness, and the newborn's sensory-motor skills. Parents are helped to understand that their newborn is making a transition to life outside the womb while learning what to expect from the world through experiences with caregivers (Brazelton & Cramer, 1990).

The postpartum period is an opportune time to teach new parents because they are highly motivated learners. Both formal and informal educational opportunities are important. Teaching and role modeling infant care mainly takes place while providing bedside care for mother and baby, but group teaching sessions can reinforce and increase the bedside learning by demonstrating other babies' unique characteristics. Group teaching sessions are not only time efficient but also provide an opportunity for discussion, exchange of ideas, mutual problem solving, and group support.

Breastfeeding

The World Health Organization (WHO), the American Academy of Pediatrics (AAP), the American College of Obstetricians and Gynecologists (ACOG), and the Association of Women's Health, Obstetrics and Neonatal Nurses (AWHONN) all have endorsed breastfeeding as the preferred method of feeding in the first year of life (American Academy of Pediatrics, 1997; Kyenkya-Isabirye, 1992; Saadeh & Akre, 1996).

In 1991, the United Nation's Children's Fund (UNICEF) and WHO developed the Baby Friendly Hospital Initiative as part of a worldwide program. Its ultimate goal is to assure that all babies worldwide are breastfed (Kyenkya-Isabirye, 1992).

Maternity and pediatric programs can be designated as "baby friendly" by implementing the Initiative's 10 Steps to Successful Breastfeeding (Box 2-1). SRMC programs often strive to achieve this designation.

BOX 2–1

Ten Steps to Successful Breastfeeding

Every facility providing maternity services and care for newborn infants should:

1. Have a written breastfeeding policy that is routinely communicated to all healthcare staff.
2. Train all healthcare staff in skills necessary to implement this policy.
3. Inform all pregnant women about the benefits and management of breastfeeding.
4. Help mothers initiate breastfeeding within a half-hour of birth.
5. Show mothers how to breastfeed, and how to maintain lactation even if they should be separated from their infants.
6. Give newborn infants no food or drink other than breast milk, unless *medically* indicated.
7. Practice rooming-in—allow mothers and infants to remain together—24 hours a day.
8. Encourage breastfeeding on demand.
9. Give no artificial teats or pacifiers (also called dummies or soothers) to breastfeeding infants.
10. Foster the establishment of breastfeeding support groups and refer mothers to them on discharge from the hospital or clinic.

(From The Global Criteria for the WHO/UNICEF Baby Friendly Hospital Initiative, March 1992.)

Discharge and Home Follow-Up

At the time of discharge from the hospital, the nurse gives each family specific, written information that reinforces hospital teaching. The discharge packet includes information about community resources that may be useful, such as parent-baby support groups, breastfeeding support groups, parenting classes, and mother-to-mother volunteer programs. Written material should be appropriately targeted to the family's needs—for example, for teens or low-literacy families—and it should be in the native language of limited or non-English speakers.

At a minimum, the hospital provides a "warmline" that new parents can easily call to get questions answered or information on infant care. Optimal programs also provide either home visits or return visits. Postpartum home or return visits include both physical and psychosocial evaluation of mother and baby as well as a breastfeeding evaluation.

Postpartum parent groups and breastfeeding support groups are formed for ongoing support of families. In addition, the organization works with community agencies to create a safety net for families at risk.

Grief

SRMC programs also have formal bereavement services for grieving families. All staff members receive training to help grieving families. There are many opportunities to develop a grief counseling team. Interested and committed staff members can be supported to become certified grief counselors. These specially prepared staff, along with representatives of social services and pastoral care, can comprise a grief counseling team, whose primary objective is to console the grieving family in the hospital. The team also provides ongoing support in the form of phone follow-up and bereavement counseling.

SUMMARY

SRMC is a care program and facility plan that was designed to facilitate the provision of socially responsive maternity care. Day-to-day care embodies the philosophy and operating principles of family-centered maternity care. All members of the clinical staff promote SRMC goals and further them in every interaction with every member of the childbearing families they serve. This requires a level and scope of practice that goes beyond conventional medical and nursing care.

REFERENCES

American Academy of Pediatrics (1997). Work group on breastfeeding. Breastfeeding and the use of human milk. *Pediatrics, 100*(6), 1035–1039.

American Academy of Pediatrics Task Force on Circumcision (1999). Circumcision policy statement. *Pediatrics, 103*(3), 686.

Association of Women's Health, Obstetric and Neonatal Nurses (1998). *Standards and guidelines for professional nursing practice in the care of women and newborns* (5th ed.). Washington, D.C.: Author.

Biancuzzo, M. (1995). Six myths of maternal posture during labor. *Maternal Child Nursing Journal, 18,* 264–269.

Biancuzzo, M. (1999). The breastfeeding advisor: Nursing the preterm baby. *Childbirth Instructor Magazine, 8,* 10–11.

Brazelton, T.B., & Cramer, B.G. (1990). *The earliest relationship: Parents, infants, and the drama of early attachment.* Reading, MA: Addison-Wesley.

Bryanton, J., Fraser-Davey, H., & Sullivan, P. (1994). Women's perceptions of nursing support during labor. *Journal of Obstetric, Gynecologic, and Neonatal Nursing, 23*(8), 638–644.

Canadian Institute of Child Health (1996). *National breastfeeding guidelines for health care providers* (rev.). Ottawa, Canada: Canadian Institute of Child Health.

Carty, E.M., & Tier, T. (1989). Birth planning: A reality-based script for building confidence. *Journal of Nurse-Midwifery, 34*(3), 111–114.

Cogan, R., & Spinnato, J.A. (1988). Social support during premature labor: Effects on labor and the newborn. *Journal of Psychosomatic Obstetrics and Gynaecology, 8,* 209–216.

Doulas of North America (1998). Position paper: The doula's contribution to modern maternity care. *International Doula, 6*(3), 14–17.

Fowles, E.R. (1998). Labor concerns of women two months after delivery. *Birth, 25*(4), 235–240.

Frede, D.J., & Strohbach, M.E. (1992). The state of preconceptual health education. *Journal of Perinatal Education, 9*(2), 19–26.

Gagnon, A.J., Waghorn, K., & Covell, C. (1997). A randomized trial of one-to-one nurse support of women in labor. *Birth, 24*(2), 71–77.

Gagnon, A., & Waghorn, K. (1996). Supportive care by maternity nurses: A work sampling study in an intrapartum unit. *Birth, 23*(1), 1–6.

The global criteria for the WHO/UNICEF Baby Friendly Hospital Initiative (1992). *UNICEF Guidelines.*

Goer, H. (1989). The fascinating world of the unborn. *Reader's Digest,* November, 150–154.

Goer, H. (1991). Not just another way to have a baby. *Baby Talk,* November, 34–35, 41, 61.

Gordon, N.P., Walton, D., McAdam, E., Derman, J., Gallitero, G., & Garrett, L. (1999). Effects of providing hospital-based doulas in health maintenance organization hospitals. *Obstetrics and Gynecology, 93,* 422–466.

Grunwald, P.C., & Becker, P.T. (1990). Developmental enhancement: Implementing a program for the NICU. *Neonatal Network, 9*(6), 29–30, 39–45.

Hodnett, E. (1996). Nursing support of the laboring woman. *Journal of Obstetric, Gynecologic, and Neonatal Nursing, 25*(3), 257–264.

Hodnett, E.D. (1999). Caregiver support for women during childbirth (Cochrane Review). In *The Cochrane Library*, Issue 1. Oxford: Update Software.

Hodnett, E.D., & Osborn, W. (1989). Effects of continuous intrapartum professional support on childbirth outcomes. *Research in Nursing and Health, 12*, 289–297.

Humenick, S.S. (1981). Mastery: The key to childbirth satisfaction? A review. *Birth, 8*(2), 79–83.

Humenick, S.S., & Bugen, L.A. (1981). Mastery: The key to childbirth satisfaction? A study. *Birth, 8*(2), 84–89.

Kennell, J., Klaus, M., McGrath, S., Robertson, S., & Hinkley, C. (1991). Continuous emotional support during labor in a US hospital. *JAMA, 265*(17), 2197–2201.

Kennell, J., & McGrath, S.K. (1993). Labor support by a doula for middle income couples: The effect on cesarean rates. *Pediatric Research, 33*, 12A.

Klaus, M.H., Kennell, J.H., & Klaus, P.H. (1995). *Bonding: Building the foundations of secure attachment and independence.* Reading, MA: Addison-Wesley.

Klaus, M.H., Kennell, J.H., Robertson, S.S., & Sosa, R. (1986). Effects of social support during parturition on maternal and infant morbidity. *British Medical Journal, 293*, 585–587.

Kuhn, J. (1984). Updating family-centered maternity care: Application of a conceptual analysis of support. *Health Care of Women International, 5*, 93–101.

Kyenkya-Isabirye, M. (1992). UNICEF launches the baby-friendly hospital initiative. *Maternal Child Nursing Journal, 17*, 177–179.

Losch, M., Dungy, C.I., Russell, D., & Dusdieker, L.B. (1995). Impact of attitudes on maternal decisions regarding infant feeding. *Journal of Pediatrics, 126*(4), 507–512.

Madi, B.C., Sandall, J., Bennett, R., & McLeod, C. (1999). Effects of female relative support in labor: A randomized controlled trial. *Birth, 26*(1), 4–8.

Martin, S., Landry, S., Steelman, L., Kennell, J. H., & McGrath, S. (1998). The effect of doula support during labor on mother-infant interaction at 2 months. *Infant Behavioral Development, 21*(Suppl), 556.

McNiven, P., Hodnett, E.D., & O'Brien-Pallas, L. (1992). Supporting women in labor: A work sampling study of the activities of labor and delivery nurses. *Birth, 19*(1), 3–8.

Mead, M. (1965). *Family*. New York: Macmillan.

Perez, P., & Snedeker, C. (1990). *Special women: The role of the professional labor assistant.* Johnson, VT: Cutting Edge Press.

Phillips, C. (1994). *Family-centered maternity care.* Minneapolis: International Childbirth Education Association, Inc.

Phillips, C.R. (1997). *Mother-baby nursing.* Washington, D.C.: Association of Women's Health, Obstetric and Neonatal Nurses.

Raisler, J., & O'Campo, P. (1999). Breastfeeding and infant illness: A dose-response relationship? *American Journal of Public Health, 89*(1), 25–29.

Saadeh, R., & Akre, T. (1996). Ten steps to successful breastfeeding: A summary of the rationale and scientific evidence. *Birth, 23*(3), 154–160.

Simkin, P. (1991). Just another day in a woman's life? Women's long-term perceptions of their first birth experience. Part I. *Birth, 18*(4), 203–210.

Simkin, P.T. (1992). Just another day in a woman's life? Part II: Nature and consistency of women's long-term memories of their first birth experiences. *Birth, 19*(2), 64–81.

Simpson, K.R., & Knox, G.E. (1999). Strategies for developing an evidence-based aprpoach to perinatal care. *American Journal of Maternal/Child Nursing, 24*(3), 122–131.

Tarka, M.T., & Paunonen, M. (1996). Social support and its impact on mothers' experiences of childbirth. *Journal of Advanced Nursing, 23*(1), 70–75.

Todd, L. (1998). Reciprocal interactions as the foundation for parent-infant attachment. *International Journal of Childbirth Education, 13*(4), 5–8.

Tomlinson, P.S., Mattson Bryan, A.A., & Lash Esau, A. (1996). Family-centered intrapartum care: Revisiting an old concept. *Journal of Obstetric, Gynecologic, and Neonatal Nursing, 25*(4), 331–337.

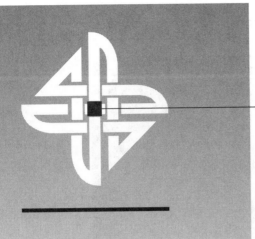

CHAPTER 3

Professional Practice in Single-Room Maternity Care

PROFESSIONAL PRACTICE IN SRMC

Whether it is a startup program or a transition from a multitransfer system (either with delivery or LDR rooms), creating successful SRMC is primarily a process of program and practice development. Through our experience over the past 2 decades, we have come to recognize that success depends primarily on people and processes and much less on facility. Before committing to SRMC facility design, the organization must understand what is involved in creating an excellent SRMC program. Quite simply, it is not advisable to embark on either facility or program development unless medical and nursing staffs understand and are willing to deliver the SRMC program of care.

CLINICAL CARE IN SRMC

Professional practice in SRMC is different in important respects from conventional obstetric medical and nursing care. Clinical care in SRMC focuses on pregnancy as a "normal" condition. Family, not hospital or staff needs, are priority; care is organized and delivered in the context of the family; and families are involved in the care process.

FAMILY EDUCATION

A prerequisite for effective family development is a community education program that begins as early as possible, preferably before conception. SRMC programs integrate community and prenatal care into the operation of the clinical services in order to meet their goals. A comprehensive community and childbirth education and parenting program helps parents-to-be to make healthful choices about conception, pregnancy, childbirth, and infant care (Biasella, 1993). This, in turn, helps to achieve the desired outcomes of healthy mothers and healthy babies, capable mothers and fathers who can parent, and family development (Figure 3-1).

Those choices that relate to health maintenance, breastfeeding, nutrition, preparation for normalcy-oriented labor and birth, pain relief, and cessation or avoidance of harmful agents will directly affect maternal and infant health outcomes. Teaching about these issues is comprehensive and adapted to the needs of each woman and her family. Clinicians integrate clinical care with education about that care throughout the childbearing year.

It is necessary for childbirth educators to understand the principles and practice of physiologic labor and birth support. Prenatal education can help make families comfortable with this concept and teaches techniques families can

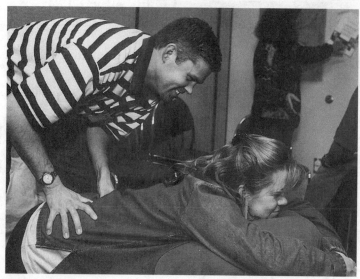

FIGURE 3–1. Childbirth and parenting education. (Photo courtesy of the Family Maternity Center, Evergreen Hospital, Kirkland, WA.)

use to make labor more comfortable and productive.

Maternity care providers and staff must be knowledgeable about the content of prenatal and parenting education programs so there is a seamless integration with clinical practice. For the same reason, educators should be knowledgeable about clinical and nursing programs. This shared knowledge is best achieved when childbirth and community educators also serve in the maternity unit as nurses, monitrices, or doulas, and when providers such as physicians and midwives play an active role in the education programs.

Physiologic Management of Labor and Birth

Since earliest recorded history, women of all cultures have used positioning as a way to make labor and birth quicker, easier, and more comfortable (Englemann, 1977). Restrictions on the mother's ability to use her body result in prolonged, painful, or unproductive labor, thus increasing the need for assisted instrumental or cesarean delivery. These interventions can affect the woman's postpartum course, her ability to nurture her newborn, and her overall childbirth experience. Few women in America today experience physiologic birthing, and many have no expectation that it is possible.

Maternal positioning, and especially freedom to change from one position to another, assist the labor's progress in a number of different ways. Spinal flexion produced by leaning forward from a standing or sitting position, or by curling forward from a lying position, reduces the lumbar curve, thus smoothing out the S-shaped path that the baby's head would otherwise take around the pubis (Figure 3-2).

Three generations of conventional American obstetric and newborn care have buried the expectations and skills needed to empower women to birth their babies. Fortunately, women have not lost the innate urge to respond to discomfort in labor by adopting positions that are helpful to the baby's passage. A study conducted in a major teaching hospital showed that, even in a group whose cultural expectation is that one lies in bed in labor, women still responded to labor by position changes when allowed to do so and used physiologic positioning to relieve the discomfort of labor (Figure 3-3). Even when not instructed in the benefits of movement, but when simply permitted to move freely, laboring women changed position an average of 7.5 times (Carlson, Diel, Sachtelben-Murray, McRae, Fenwick & Friedman, 1986).

When supine or standing, the plane of the human pelvic brim is not perpendicular to the spinal axis. Spinal flexion reduces the lumbar curve, providing the fetus with a straighter path through the birth canal.

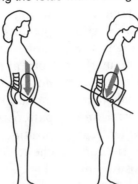

FIGURE 3–2. Spinal flexion reduces the lumbar curve, providing the fetus with a straighter path through the birth canal.

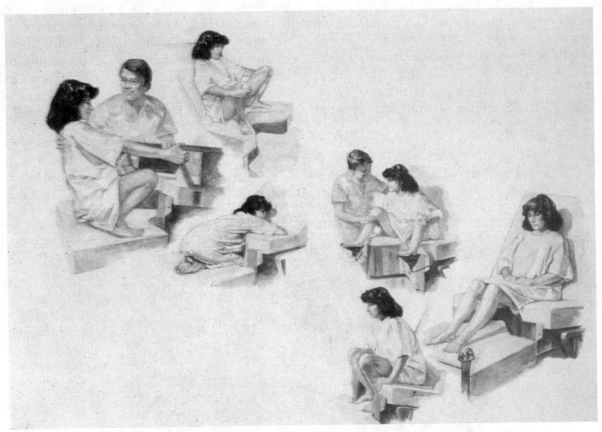

FIGURE 3–3. When permitted to move freely, laboring women change position frequently.

A true upright position, as contrasted to a reclining or supine position, allows the uterus to fall forward, away from the mother's spine. Besides causing maternal hypotension, compression of the inferior vena cava, and possible fetal distress, the supine position also misaligns the uterus with the pelvic inlet. By tipping the uterus forward, a sitting or standing position increases the angle between the uterus and maternal spine, improving alignment with the pelvic brim and directing the presenting part into the wider, rear part of the pelvis (Gold, 1950; Figure 3-4). Studies have demonstrated that upright positioning shortens the duration of the first and second stages of labor (Caldyro-Barcia, 1979; Diaz, Schwarcz, Fescina & Caldyro-Barcia, 1980; Liu, 1989; Roberts, Mendez-Bauer & Woodell, 1983). Although recent studies (Goer, 1999) do not support earlier findings that walking shortens duration of labor, they do indicate that walking allows a woman to feel more in control without causing any harm.

Upright positions also produce stronger expulsive forces in labor as a result of a reflex stimulated by pressure on the lower birth canal. Gravity adds 10 to 35 mmHg of additional pressure to the presenting part (Caldyro-Barcia, 1979; Read, Miller & Paul, 1981), and contractions are longer, stronger, and more frequent when the woman is upright. In addition, upright women produce lower levels of stress-related hormones (beta-endorphin, ACTH, cortisol, and epinephrine) than do supine women. The well-documented labor-inhibiting effects of these hormones may be associated with dystotic labor patterns (Fenwick & Simkin, 1987). In an upright position, the woman can freely use her arm, chest, and abdominal muscles to birth her baby (Figure 3-5). Side-lying can also be comforting and effective for labor and pushing.

No single position is ideal for all stages of the baby's travel through the maternal pelvis. The relationship between the presenting part and the pelvis is often not optimal due to asynclitism, deflexion, or occipito-posterior presentation of the baby's head. This is commonly associated with pain, which the unrestricted woman may try to relieve by position changes. This offers a greater variety of angles to the presenting part, increasing the chance of a better fit between baby and pelvis (Fenwick & Simkin, 1987; Figure 3-6). Position changes have been shown to be helpful

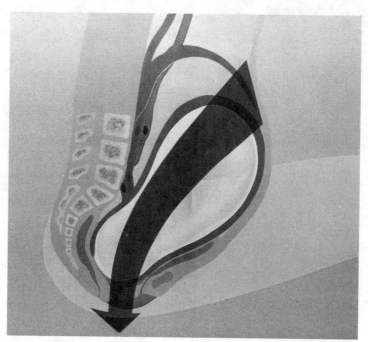

FIGURE 3–4. A true upright position tips the uterus forward, away from the mother's spine.

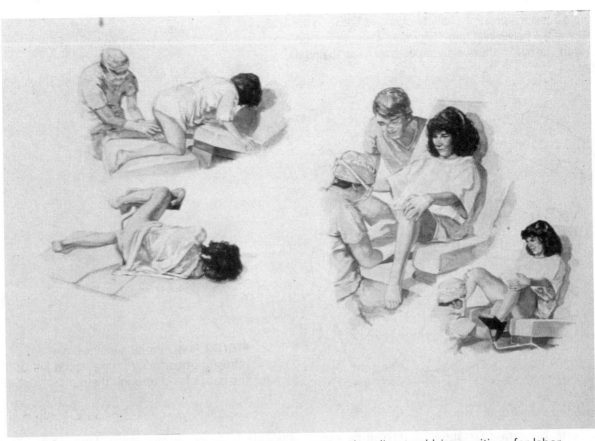

FIGURE 3–5. Women have always chosen sitting, squatting, kneeling, and lying positions for labor and birth.

in rotating the fetal head from a posterior to an anterior position (Andrews & Andrews, 1983; Figure 3-7).

During labor, maternal position changes are encouraged by the mother's caregivers and are facilitated by showing women how to use labor aids such as a squatting bar, a "birthing ball," room furniture, or even her coach's body. Figure 3-8 demonstrates how a birthing ball and birth bed can help support labor and birth positioning.

The pelvis' ability to change shape is seldom recognized or put to beneficial use in labor management. The joint-softening effects of the hormone relaxin allow an increase in the woman's pelvis capacity up to 30% over that produced by walking or squatting (Borell & Fernstrom, 1966; Russell, 1969) (Figure 3-9). Sitting upright on a chair or pressure from sitting on the ischial tuberosities also widen separation of the ischial bones. To birth in this position requires a birthing bed that has an opening for birth. To birth a baby over a straight edge, the mother must first lie back. This removes the forces that separate her ischia and decreases her pelvis's antero-posterior diameter by transferring her weight to her sacrum (Fenwick & Simkin, 1987). Positioning is also important in managing malpresentations such as occipito-posterior presentation of the baby's head and fetal distress associated with supine hypotension.

Maternal Pushing Efforts

Valsalva maneuvers and prolonged bearing-down effort produce a fall in maternal cardiac output and are associated with a decrease in placental circulation and an increase in fetal hypoxia (McKay, 1980; Roberts & Woolley, 1996).

Multiple positions present a variety of angles between the fetal head and the pelvic inlet, providing more chances to help the deflexed, asynclitic, transverse or posterior head to find the "right fit."

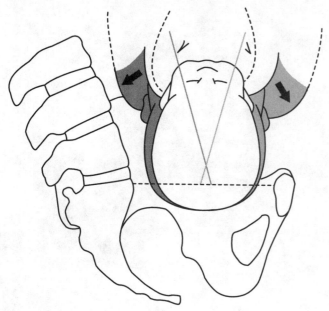

FIGURE 3–6. Position changes present different opportunities for a "good fit" of the baby's head through the mother's pelvis.

In spite of data that show that routine episiotomy is not helpful (Banta & Thacker, 1982), this is still a popular procedure among most obstetricians. One reason is that, until techniques for preventing perineal tearing have been mastered, tears occur with frequency. Techniques for preventing perineal tearing include avoiding zealous Valsalva expulsive efforts, stretching the perineum and pelvic floor ahead of the fetal head, and controlling the fetal head

Figure 1. In occipito-posterior presentations, the fetal spine intersects the fetal skull near the center of resistance. This keeps the head extended in the wide occipito-frontal diameter, preventing rotation.

Figure 2. Flexing the maternal spine redirects the downward force transmitted by the fetal spine to a point posterior to the center of resistance, flexing the head and making rotation more likely.

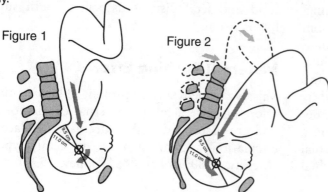

Figure 1

Figure 2

FIGURE 3–7. In occipito-posterior presentations, curling forward flexes the infant's neck, making rotation more likely.

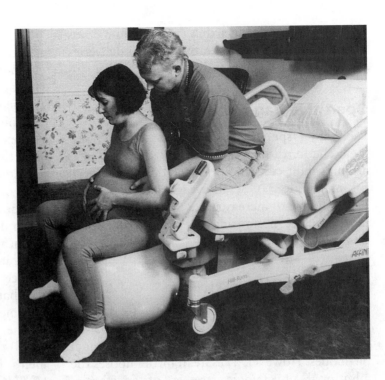

FIGURE 3–8. Birthing balls and beds designed for physiologic birth help support labor and birth positioning. (Photo courtesy of Hill-Rom, Batesville, IN.)

and shoulders during birth. In addition, flexion of the baby's head ensures that the smallest diameter, the suboccipitobregmatic, passes through the introitus. Extension of the baby's head before the nape of the neck is born, as is done in the Ritgen maneuver, will increase this diameter by more than a centimeter and increase the chance of laceration. Successful delivery of the head is often followed by a tear from delivering the shoulders. Delivering the anterior arm

completely before delivering the posterior shoulder prevents stretching the introitus by both shoulders (Fenwick, 1984).

With physiologic management of labor and birth, the woman can gain maximum benefit from her inherent physical and psychosocial resources.

When the flow of the natural labor and birth process is interrupted by fear, immobilization, medications, and other agents, it can start a "clin-

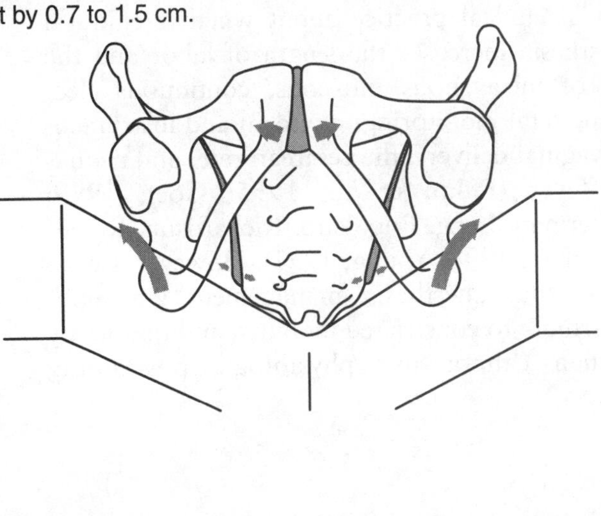

The joint-softening effects of relaxin allow the pelvis to hinge open at the pubic and sacro-iliac joints. Pressure (through sitting) on the ischial tuberosities increases the size of the pelvic outlet by 0.7 to 1.5 cm.

FIGURE 3–9. The joint-softening effects of relaxin allow the pelvis to hinge open at the pubic and sacro-iliac joints.

ical cascade" of changes that results in numerous interventions such as operative vaginal deliveries and unnecessary cesarean births.

Operative Vaginal Deliveries

Facilitating spontaneous birth through physiologic childbirth management as just described is an important consideration in reducing the need for interventions. Operative vaginal deliveries can be costly due to increased use of supplies and the need for close monitoring by nursing staff, which drives up staffing costs.

Cesarean Birth

Despite the emotional connotations of cesareans for mothers and families, a cesarean signals the beginning of a new family unit just as a vaginal birth does. However, a cesarean birth imposes the additional physiologic stresses of anesthesia, major surgery, physical recovery, and postoperative complications, including infections. In addition, when a family has prepared for a vaginal birth, an unexpected cesarean may provoke feelings of anger, disappointment, and guilt in the family members. A combination of the new mother's physical and emotional states can pose difficulties with her initial attempts to hold and feed her baby and learn about infant care.

Anesthesiology Practices in SRMC

The popularity of epidural techniques has contributed to the use of horizontal positions because women typically remain in bed from the time of administration through delivery (Shermer & Raines, 1997). Controversy exists in the literature and in clinical practice about whether epidural anesthesia increases the length of labor and the use of intravenous infusions, continuous electronic fetal monitoring, oxytocin and instrumental vaginal delivery, the cesarean rate, and neonatal fever (Enkin et al., 1995; Goer, 1999; Lieberman, Lang, Frigoletto, Richardson, Ringer & Cohen, 1997; Young, 1997). However, we do know that anesthesia management guidelines contribute to constricted mobility, and that many women cannot use physiologic positioning because of lack of mobility and strength in their legs.

Controversy also exists about the reason for the large number of epidurals given to American women. Some people believe that the current generation of childbearing women values technology and expediency and wants high-tech support and effortless labor and birth (Granninger & McCool, 1998). Others believe that the community of childbearing families has been sold on epidural anesthesia because a hospital maternity program that institutes an epidural service economically requires a large volume of epidurals to generate the payment needed to be a profitable service.

Whatever the reason, epidural analgesia has become the norm for many maternity services in the United States (Granninger & McCool, 1998). Findings from the Association of Women's Health, Obstetric and Neonatal Nurses (AWHONN) National Research Utilization Project on Second-Stage Labor Management showed that epidural rates were 50% or more in 60% of the sites surveyed, with a range from 15% to 91% (Shermer & Raines, 1997).

In our experience nationwide, there is a wide variance in skill and techniques of hospital anesthesia teams.

In some situations, the goal of labor epidural analgesia is to provide pain relief with minimal motor blockade that allows for effective pushing and, in some cases, ambulation (walking epidurals). With the adjunctive use of narcotic agents, lower concentrations and smaller doses of local anesthetic have been shown to achieve adequate pain relief while preserving the ability to use upright positions for labor and birth (Shermer & Raines, 1997). In other situations, the goal seems to be use of complete anesthesia to eliminate pain, sensation, and motor function. Obviously, a woman's ability to position herself and push effectively in second-stage labor will be affected differently in each of these situations. Epidural administration techniques that maintain the pushing effort appear to have the least impact on second-stage outcomes, including duration and need for assisted delivery (Dickinson & Naughton, 1996). New analgesic approaches such as intrathecal narcotic (ITN) analgesia or a combined spinal/epidural technique allow the woman to participate actively in labor and birth. Some of these patients are able to walk and position themselves as they desire for second-stage labor (Shermer & Raines, 1997).

Routine use of epidural analgesia for labor and vaginal birth has significant implications for hospital resources. To begin with, the use of epidural analgesia requires a one-to-one nurse-to-patient ratio for initiating epidural analgesia (American Academy of Pediatrics [AAP] & American College of Obstetricians and Gynecologists [ACOG], 1997) and close monitoring thereafter (AWHONN, 1998; AWHONN, 1996). For nonepidural patients, one-to-one staffing is not required until women enter active phase labor (AAP & ACOG, 1997). In addition to close labor monitoring, patients in the postanesthesia period should be continually observed and monitored by methods appropriate to their postpartum condition (AWHONN, 1998). This, too, affects staffing patterns and leads to higher staffing costs (Eakes, 1990). Phillips+Fenwick has worked with many hospitals where the anesthesiologist monitors the epidural from start to finish. This means that anesthesia departments need extra staff both to cover the maternity unit and to cover cesarean section rooms and main operating rooms at the same time.

Although epidural analgesia, when skillfully provided, is a valuable tool with a legitimate place in managing pain on a selected basis, there is no scientific evidence for its routine application (Enkin et al., 1995). Its routine application means that hundreds of thousands of American women receive epidurals when they could do as well or better with other types of pain management. This has a significant financial price tag. In addition, a significant number of mothers and babies are put at risk for potential complications from epidural administration.

Balancing pain relief with nonintervention in an era when it is a social norm to deliver with an epidural is a true challenge. Until more data are available, it behooves each maternity program to present clear benefits and risks of epidural analgesia/anesthesia to all childbearing families so women can make educated decisions regarding pain relief in labor. It is extremely important to teach women that there are other alternatives to pain relief in labor. Research over 2 decades has produced compelling evidence of the positive impact that labor support can have on helping to decrease the length of labor, the need for pain medications or epidurals, the need for interventions such as inductions, the use of forceps or vacuum extractors, and the cesarean birth rate (Enkin et al., 1995). Nursing staff must be able to articulate the value of one-to-one care when labor gets tough as clearly as the anesthesiologist can articulate the value of epidurals for pain relief.

The bottom line is that routine and unnecessary practices not found efficacious in delivering appropriate maternity care have a significant negative impact on profitability because they increase use of staff and supplies (Traynor & Peaceman, 1998). SRMC provides a framework for evaluating current practices and proposing improved practices.

CLINICAL CARE AFTER BIRTH

In SRMC, clinical care after birth goes beyond focusing on nonseparation of mothers and babies to include the well-being of the entire family. Medical and nursing staff are concerned about the family's adjustment to childbearing and transition to parenthood, not only during the hospital stay but also during the early weeks at home.

Mother–Baby Care

Mother–baby care is a collaborative practice model based on collegial relationships among nurses and physicians who provide maternity and newborn care. It provides many benefits to parents, hospitals, and staff (Boxes 3-1 through 3-3). This model derives from the belief, fundamental to the family-centered maternity care philosophy, that mothers and babies benefit from being together in the first hours and days of life. In mother–baby care, sometimes called couplet or dyad care, physicians and nurses perform all examinations and provide all care in the mother's room. Separating mother and infant is avoided except for brief periods during which family

BOX 3 – 1

Benefits of Mother–Baby Nursing to Family and Baby

- Provides an environment for the parents to learn about their baby's responses and sleep–wake cycles.
- Facilitates earlier establishment of biologic rhythms with flexible feeding and sleeping according to individual baby's needs.
- Helps mother sleep better with baby at her side.
- Fosters successful breastfeeding and, thus, aids in postpartum involution.
- Decreases incidence of infant cross-infection.
- Provides individualized, one-to-one attention.
- Promotes the mother's role and bonding and attachment.
- Increases educational opportunities.
- Fosters continuity of care and reduction of confusion of messages between caregivers.
- Promotes the mother's learning about her infant and self-care capabilities.
- Increases maternal self-confidence in caring for her infant.
- Eliminates anxiety about whether the baby is receiving proper care. Mother knows quality of care because she sees it.
- Maintains high patient care standards.

From Harvey, 1982; Keefe, 1987; Mansell, 1984; Norr, Roberts & Freese, 1989; Panwar, 1986; Vestal, 1982; Watters, 1985; Watters & Kristiansen, 1995; Wilkerson & Barrow, 1988.

BOX 3 – 2

Benefits of Mother–Baby Nursing to the Staff

- Increases skills and knowledge base, thus making nurses more marketable.
- Diversifies skills.
- Streamlines responsibilities for care and teaching.
- Increases nursing value to the hospital.
- Increases nurses' personal involvement and responsibility for patient care and self-learning.
- Increases accountability.
- Improves communication between family and caregivers.
- Replaces fragmented care with continuity of care.
- Eliminates duplication of services.
- Facilitates discharge planning.
- Increases efficiency and productivity.
- Improves interdisciplinary communication and teamwork.
- Increases job satisfaction through the provision of individualized care.
- Provides a more stimulating work environment.
- Elicits positive comments from families.
- Enhances image in the community due to family observation of professional skills.

From Harvey, 1982; Keefe, 1987; Mansell, 1984; Norr, Roberts & Freese, 1989; Panwar, 1986; Vestal, 1982; Watters, 1985; Watters & Kristiansen, 1995; Wilkerson & Barrow, 1988.

members provide infant care, if possible. Infant care physicians make daily rounds and perform newborn examinations in mothers' rooms. One nurse cares jointly for a postpartum mother and her newborn, and each mother–baby pair is considered a single unit. Each nurse cares for three or four mother–baby couples depending on their acuity (Phillips, 1997).

In addition to facilitating the attachment process, mother–baby nursing focuses on teaching and role modeling. Physicians, nurses, and students examine babies in the mother's room at her bedside, taking advantage of the opportunity to teach the mother and other family members. The mother–baby nurse also teaches while providing bedside care (AWHONN, 1998). Physicians and nurses use assessment skills that allow them to identify and understand each woman's attitudes, behaviors, values, and needs. Plans for care are implemented that are consistent with the new family's needs and values. In this way, mother–baby care can be provided for families with varying physical, social, and cultural needs.

BOX 3 - 3

Benefits of Mother–Baby Nursing to the Hospital

- Eliminates unnecessary rules and enhances support of justified institutional policies.
- Increases openness between community and hospital in assessing institutional quality and commitment to care.
- Improves image in the community.
- Increases favor for preventive approach to care for managed care contracts.
- Reduces nursing staff turnover through job enrichment.
- Increases staff productivity and flexibility and reduces costs.
- Adapts easily to individual family needs.
- Increases patient satisfaction.

From Harvey, 1982; Keefe, 1987; Mansell, 1984; Norr, Roberts & Freese, 1989; Panwar, 1986; Vestal, 1982; Watters, 1985; Watters & Kristiansen, 1995; Wilkerson & Barrow, 1988.

Mother–baby care differs significantly from other infant care arrangements that may allow mothers to have their infants with them in their rooms for periods of time during the day, or in which postpartum nurses care for families and nursery nurses care for babies. Further, mother–baby care is an option even for mothers who are unable to accept full responsibility for the care of their newborns, because qualified nurses provide infant care in the family's room (Phillips, 1997).

In SRMC programs, physicians and nurses do not just allow mothers to keep their babies with them, but actively encourage them to do so at all times. Two important concepts guide the practice of mother–baby care in SRMC programs. The first is that the work of parent–infant attachment in the first hours, days, and weeks of life is almost completely sensory in nature. Attachment work is what parents and babies do to get to know one another, to form a relationship that is specific and will endure across time (Figure 3-10). Attachment is always a work in progress, needing to be retooled as parents and infants grow and change. In the hours and days after birth, all senses (tactile, auditory, olfactory, visual, and taste) of both parent and infant are brought to attachment work. Because the attachment process is reciprocal, parent and infant must be together for this work to progress in a healthy manner.

The second guiding concept of mother–baby care is that for the infant, behavior is language. When assisting parents to learn to care for their infant, instructing them about infant behavior opens a door to appreciating the infant's ability to guide the parents to the infant's needs. Demon-

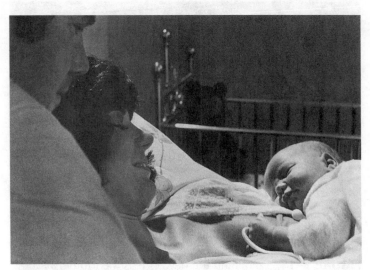

FIGURE 3–10. Attachment work is the work that parents and babies do to get to know one another.

strating newborn sensory-motor skills and giving meaning to them alerts parents to the multiple ways that infants, from birth, are active participants in a two-way conversation. Helping parents both see and experience infant state-related behavior makes the unpredictable infant more predictable. Mother–baby nursing provides one ideal forum for such education (Todd, 1998).

Separating parent and infant for any reason challenges attachment work. Parents and infants are resilient and can recover from such challenges, but asking this of them should not be done without good clinical reasons. Because mother–baby care is provided for both infant and mother, they can remain together even if the mother is not able to get out of bed. If necessary, the baby can be taken to a holding area or "respite" nursery for brief periods of time. It is not necessary to maintain a central nursery in a mother–baby program.

Location of Newborn Examination by Infant Care Provider

One pediatric practice that is typical of care provided in multitransfer models impinges on SRMC. This practice involves examining the newborn in a nursery area, away from the mother and her family. Although time-efficient for the pediatrician in the short-term, this practice interferes with an important opportunity to enhance relationships with the mother, father, and their support system, and to build their confidence and competence in knowing and caring for the infant.

Separating newborns from their mothers during pediatric rounds and for examinations increases the amount of time hospital staff members must spend transporting well babies between mothers' rooms and a separate location where the babies are examined. When postpartum and nursery nurses are educated to provide all care for both mother and baby in the mother's room, the increased efficiency can translate into dollar savings.

Examining the newborn in the mother's room presents opportunities to develop or enhance a relationship with the mother and father and the support persons important to them. This hospital experience can make or break a relationship with the pediatric care provider. Dissatisfaction with the behavior of pediatric care providers or with the quality of interaction causes many parents to change providers after leaving the hospital. On the other hand, good experiences in the hospital lead to informed choice of the baby's doctor.

The physician and nurse can teach parents and other family members about normal newborn behavior, reactions, and physiology (Figure 3-11).

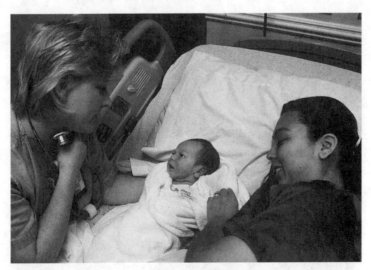

FIGURE 3–11. Examining the newborn in the mother's room. (Photo courtesy of Dartmouth-Hitchcock Medical Center, Lebanon, NH.)

This learning can improve the observational skills of the parents and other family members as well as reinforce the bond between the baby and the parents. In addition, the physician can model handling and examining an infant, which also benefits parents and other family members.

This early investment in relationships and parent teaching saves time for the infant care provider in the end. Having mothers who are more knowledgeable and families who feel comfortable and confident with their physician can reduce unnecessary calls and healthcare expenditures. In addition, meeting families at the bedside and demonstrating competent and compassionate care can increase consumer satisfaction. Consumer satisfaction leads to referrals.

Physicians may be concerned that examining the newborn in the mother's room will take excess time, keeping them away from their office practices longer than necessary. They may also have concerns about adequate lighting and having appropriate equipment to do a thorough examination in the mother's room. Some pediatric physicians worry that it will be difficult if an abnormality is discovered in the parents' presence, and they express reluctance and discomfort about how best to share this information with new parents.

Contrary to these fears about dealing with problems in the presence of family, parents prefer being told the "bad news" early and together by physicians who are actually in physical contact with their baby. Physicians being available and providing medical information and support are important to bereaved parents.

Implementing mother–baby care may require that some changes be made to allow for examining the newborn in the mother's room. Solutions to common concerns include providing a newborn examination kit for each group practice that can be stored in a convenient and safe place on the unit and providing appropriate lighting in each patient room (a ceiling spotlight of "natural" light is adequate; Beckett, Wynn & Redmond, 1996).

Implementation of Mother–Baby Care

Because mother–baby care differs from the conventional fragmented-care model, it requires reorganizing the system of postpartum and newborn care for physicians and nurses. Necessary changes can be difficult for physicians because the routine events of their traditional hospital practice are perceived to be more convenient than those required by the new model. These changes can be difficult for nurses who are accustomed to working in only one area and practicing as either postpartum or nursery nurses. With education and experience, however, most physicians and nurses find increased satisfaction in the expanded opportunities of mother–baby care.

In our experience, it is helpful to involve physicians when planning and developing new SRMC protocols to define and direct the provision of mother–baby care. This collaboration can result in the development of solutions to common concerns. New routines and procedures can be developed that support, rather than prevent, the provision of this contemporary model of care. Maternity program leadership must remain committed to making the change to bedside newborn examinations and to providing consistent, supportive leadership during the changeover.

Benefits of SRMC Nursing

In summary, SRMC nurses are educated about family-centered maternity care, becoming skilled in labor and delivery, postpartum, and newborn care. SRMC nursing offers many benefits to family development in the postpartum period. Mothers can learn to care for their babies in a supportive atmosphere with expert assistance readily available, which maximizes educational opportunities during the postpartum stay and helps prevent information overload. Examination and care of the newborn at the mother's bedside offer additional opportunities for education. Teachable moments are maximized. Discharge proceeds more smoothly because the mother is empowered throughout childbirth and the postpartum period to provide self-care and infant care under the watchful eye and careful guidance of a single nurse who has systematically integrated education and clinical care into a seamless whole. The family benefits from continuity of care. In particular, they receive more consistent information and advice. Finally, SRMC promotes breastfeeding on demand.

SRMC nursing also benefits the hospital by avoiding duplication of staff and overlap of responsibilities. This improves quality of care and helps contain costs because it makes more efficient use of the time that professionals spend providing care. It enhances nursing accountability. Professional nurses who are committed to furthering the goals of SRMC nurture families.

Provider Practice and Cost Control

Providers must appreciate their practice's impact on the use of facility, staff, and other hospital resources (Rutledge, Parsons & Bernard, 1996). Physician decisions directly affect from 70% to 90% of all US healthcare outlay (Kleinke, 1998). Excessive and unnecessary interventions cost the hospital money. When risk is shifted to physician providers in capitation contracts, the economics of eliminating excessive utilization and variability are shifted also (Kleinke, 1998).

Generally, providing maternity care on the premise that birth is natural and most intervention is unnecessary can increase profitability and productivity and can result in the highest-quality low-cost care (Simpson & Knox, 1999). Many studies show that common procedures such as routine restriction of food and fluids, routine episiotomy, and routine separation of the mother and newborn are unlikely to prove beneficial (Enkin et al., 1995). Routine continuous electronic fetal monitoring remains controversial. A large study has shown that when monitoring is routine, cesarean sections and other interventions increase without improvement in fetal outcome (Shy, Larson & Luthy, 1987). Well-designed, large-scale prospective controlled trials have not demonstrated improved fetal outcomes from the use of continuous electronic fetal monitoring (Levenco, Cunningham & Nelson, 1986), and it is suggested that fetal monitoring both decreases and increases liability to lawsuits. Fewer unnecessary interventions during labor and birth mean less equipment and supplies, medications, and lower staffing costs. Research consistently shows that interventions during labor and birth can be safely reduced (Enkin et al., 1995; Goer, 1999; Rooks, 1997; Simpson & Knox, 1999).

Normalcy-based practice is nurtured by a belief that childbirth is essentially a natural process. Certainly, childbirth is a process that can go awry, but it is, nevertheless, a process best managed by encouraging the normal instead of by treating birth as a pathologic event. Historically, most medical and nursing schools did not hold this view, and many physicians and nurses have never witnessed the normal course of spontaneous labor and birth. Educating maternity care providers and developing confidence in normalcy-based management are challenging yet essential components of implementing a successful SRMC program. In most situations, this orientation can only be achieved by a structured education program using skilled physician and nurse clinicians brought in for this purpose.

Normalcy-based professional practice in SRMC is not only best for the family, it also saves money. Facilitating spontaneous birth through physiologic childbirth management is an important consideration in reducing the need for interventions. Physicians can learn about normalcy-oriented labor and birth management and can achieve the attitudes and skills necessary to improve maternity care while at the same time reducing the high costs associated with unnecessary interventions.

Stewardship and Practice

Routine hospitalization for antepartum care, cesarean rates higher than the national average, and large numbers of scheduled procedures add significant cost to the provision of maternity care.

Antepartum Admission Rates

Ideally, SRMC programs emphasize providing antepartum care in the home to avoid hospitalization. This allows for close monitoring of clinical progress and helps ensure that the high-risk mother receives the support of her entire family to allow optimal infant attachment at the time of birth. Providing care for high-risk patients in their homes is an important consideration in promoting family attachment to the new infant while helping to minimize the financial impact.

When home care for high-risk mothers is not possible, physicians working in SRMC programs develop strategies for antepartum patients' care that allow for extensive family involvement and support for high-risk mothers. Unnecessary admissions are avoided through reliance on home-care support systems. When necessary, admissions are brief and care is focused around developing family and clinical support systems designed to make early discharge possible.

Cesarean Rates

The cesarean rate impacts the average length of stay (ALOS), which impacts facility utilization, facility costs (space), equipment requirements, supply use, and staffing. Therefore, both the mean cesarean rate for the obstetric department and individual physician cesarean rates are of critical concern when considering the financial impact of physician practice. In addition, cesarean rates are a primary quality-of-care indicator for most managed care and consumer report cards. Accreditation by the Joint Commission on Accreditation of Healthcare Organizations (JCAHO) requires submission of cesarean delivery and vaginal birth after cesarean (VBAC) data as two of the ten obstetric indicators the JCAHO monitors (Muri, 1997). The hospital's performance rate is also a factor care organizations consider when awarding contracts to hospitals and physicians. Payers' demand for demonstrable value in healthcare purchasing is causing providers to revisit the cesarean issue with new urgency.

Scheduled Procedures

Facility planners determine the necessary number of labor/delivery/recovery/postpartum (LDRP) rooms by using a calculation based largely on random occurrence of events. When providers schedule a large number of labor inductions or elective repeat cesareans at one time, there can be too many patients for the available LDRPs.

Because the priority for LDRP usage is usually given to women awaiting labor induction or cesarean birth, postpartum families may be moved from the LDRP room to another room within the facility. Moving a family to another room at this time disrupts family interaction and can create patient dissatisfaction. This move also increases the hospital's costs of patient transfer, room cleaning, and resource utilization. This problem is not unique to SRMC but also occurs in settings using delivery rooms or LDRs when large numbers of inductions or repeat cesareans are scheduled at one time.

SUMMARY

For SRMC programs to succeed, medical and nursing staff must support the philosophy that is SRMC's foundation. This requires that all practices be objectively examined to determine, through sound scientific evidence, the best approach to meeting the family's clinical, emotional, and social needs. Each procedure must be evaluated, not only in terms of its clinical effectiveness, but also as to its effects on family interaction and the development of family confidence and competence.

REFERENCES

American Academy of Pediatrics & American College of Obstetricians and Gynecologists. (1997). *Guidelines for perinatal care* (4th ed.). Elk Grove, IL: American Academy of Pediatrics.

Andrews, C. M., & Andrews, E. C. (1983). Nursing, maternal postures, and fetal position. *Nursing Research, 32*(6), 336–341.

Association of Women's Health, Obstetric and Neonatal Nurses. (1998). *Achieving consistent quality care: Using evidence to guide practice.* Washington, DC: Author.

Association of Women's Health, Obstetric and Neonatal Nurses. (1996). *Obstetrical epidural analgesia and the role of the professional registered nurse* [clinical commentary]. Washington, DC: Author.

Banta, D., & Thacker, S. (1982). Benefits and risks of episiotomy: A review. *Birth, 9*(1), 25–30.

Beckett, P., Wynn, B., & Redmond, S. (1996). Mother–baby nursing: A road map for success: Changing traditional delivery system to a single-room service. *Mother–Baby Journal, 1*(1), 7–13.

Biasella, S. (1993). A comprehensive perinatal education program. In: F. H. Nichols (Ed.), *Perinatal edu-*

cations: *AWHONN's clinical issues in perinatal and women's health nursing* (pp 5–19). Philadelphia, PA: J. B. Lippincott.

Borell, V., & Fernstrom, L. (1966). The mechanism of labor. *Radiology Clinics of North America, 5,* 73.

Caldyro-Barcia, R. (1979). The influence of maternal position on time of spontaneous rupture of the membranes, progress of labor, and fetal head compression. *Birth and the Family Journal, 6,* 17.

Carlson, J. M., Diel, J. A., Sachtelben-Murray, M., McRae, M., Fenwick, L., & Friedman, E. A. (1986). Maternal positioning during parturition in normal labor. *Obstetrics and Gynecology, 68,* 443–447.

Diaz, A. G., Schwarcz, R., Fescina, R., & Caldyro-Barcia, R. (1980). Vertical position during the first stage of the course of labor and neonatal outcome. *European Journal of Obstetrics and Gynaecology, 11*(1), 1–7.

Dickinson, B., & Naughton, N. (1996). OB anesthesiology at the University of Michigan. *The Michigan Airway, IV*(2), 1, 36.

Eakes, M. (1990). Economic considerations for epidural anesthesia in childbirth. *Nursing Economic$, 8*(5), 329–332.

Englemann, G. L. (1977). *Labor among primitive peoples* (2nd ed.). St. Louis: J. H. Chalmers and Co.

Enkin, M. (1995). Effective care in pregnancy and childbirth: The Cochrane pregnancy and childbirth database. *Journal of Perinatal Education, 4*(4), 23–25.

Fenwick, L. (1984). Birthing: Techniques for managing the physiologic and psychosocial aspects of childbirth. *Journal of Perinatology and Neonatology,* 51–62.

Fenwick, L., & Simkin, P. (1987). Maternal positioning to prevent or alleviate dystocia in labor, *Clinical Obstetrics and Gynecology. 30*(1), 83–89.

Goer, H. (1999). *The thinking woman's guide to a better birth.* New York: Perigee.

Gold, E. (1950). Pelvic drive in obstetrics: An x-ray study of 100 cases. *American Journal of Obstetrics and Gynecology, 59,* 890.

Granninger, W. M., & McCool, W. P. (1998). Nurse-midwives' use of and attitudes toward epidural analgesia. *Journal of Nurse-Midwifery, 43*(4), 250–260.

Harvey, K. (1982). Mother–baby nursing. *Nursing Management, 13*(7), 22–23.

Keefe, M. R. (1987). The impact of infant rooming-in on maternal sleep at night. *Journal of Obstetric, Gynecologic, and Neonatal Nursing, 17*(2), 122–126.

Kleinke, J. D. (1998). *Bleeding edge: The business of health care in the new century.* Gaithersburg, MD: Aspen.

Levenco, K. J., Cunningham, F. G., & Nelson, K. B. (1986). A perspective comparison of selective and universal electronic fetal monitoring in 34,995 pregnancies. *New England Journal of Medicine, 315*(10), 615–619.

Lieberman, E., Lang, J. M., Frigoletto, F., Jr., Richardson, D. K., Ringer, S. A., & Cohen, A. (1997). Epidural analgesia, intrapartum fever, and neonatal sepsis evaluation. *Pediatrics, 99*(3), 415–419.

Liu, Y. C. (1989). The effects of the upright position during childbirth. *Image: Journal of Nursing Scholarship, 21,* 14–18.

McKay, S. (1980). Maternal position during labor and birth. *Journal of Obstetric, Gynecologic, and Neonatal Nursing, 9,* 288.

Muri, J. H. (1997). The Joint Commission's ORYX initiative: Implications for perinatal nursing and care. *Journal of Perinatal Neonatal Nursing, 12*(1), 1–10.

Norr, K. F., Roberts, J. E., & Freese, U. (1989). Early postpartum rooming-in and maternal attachment behaviors in a group of medically indigent primiparas. *Journal of Nurse-Midwifery, 34,* 85–91.

Panwar, S. (1986). Introducing family-centered care for mothers and newborns. *Nursing Management, 17*(11), 45–47.

Phillips, C. R. (1997). *Mother–baby nursing.* Washington, DC: Association of Women's Health, Obstetric and Neonatal Nurses.

Read, J. A., Miller, F., & Paul, R. (1981). Randomized trial of ambulation versus oxytocin for labor enhancement: A preliminary report. *American Journal of Obstetrics and Gynecology, 139,* 669.

Roberts, J., Mendez-Bauer, C., & Woodell, D. (1983). The effects of maternal position on uterine contractibility and efficiency. *Birth, 10,* 243.

Roberts, J., & Woolley, D. (1996). A second look at the second stage of labor. *Journal of Obstetric, Gynecologic, and Neonatal Nursing, 25*(5), 415–423.

Russell, J. J. B. (1969). Moulding of the pelvic outlet. *Journal of Obstetrics and Gynecology of the British Commonwealth, 76,* 817–820.

Rutledge, R. W., Parsons, S., & Bernard, B. (1996). Cost containment strategies by private hospitals: Their effectiveness, importance, and use. *Journal of Health Care Finances, 22*(3), 1–14.

Shermer, R. H., & Raines, D. A. (1997). Positioning during the second stage of labor: Moving back to basics. *Journal of Obstetric, Gynecologic, and Neonatal Nursing, 26*(6), 727–734.

Shy, K. L., Larson, E. B., & Luthy, D. A. (1987). Evaluating a new technology: The effectiveness of electronic fetal monitoring. *Annual Review of Public Health, 8,* 165–190.

Simpson, K. R., & Knox, E. (1999). Strategies for developing an evidence-based approach to perinatal care. *MCN, The American Journal of Maternal Child Nursing, 24*(3), 122–131.

Todd, L. (1998). Reciprocal interactions as the foundation for parent–infant attachment. *International Journal of Childbirth Education, 13*(4), 5–8.

Traynor, J. D., & Peaceman, A. M. (1998). Maternal hospital charges associated with trial of labor versus elective repeat cesarean. *Birth, 25*(2), 81–84.

Vestal, K. (1982). A proposal: Primary nursing for the mother–baby dyad. *Nursing Clinics of North America, 17*(3), 3–9.

Watters, N. E. (1985). Combined mother–infant nursing care. *Journal of Obstetric, Gynecologic, and Neonatal Nursing, 14,* 478–483.

Watters, N. E., & Kristiansen, C. M. (1995). Two evaluations of combined mother–infant versus separate postnatal nursing care. *Research in Nursing and Health, 18*(1), 17–26.

Wilkerson, N. N., & Barrow, T. L. (1988). Reuniting mothers and babies: Synchronizing care with mother–baby rhythms. *MCN, The American Journal of Maternal Child Nursing, 13,* 264–268.

Young, D. (1997). Epidurals under scrutiny in the United States. *Birth, 24*(3), 139–140.

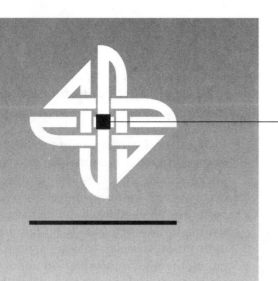

CHAPTER 4

Staff Composition and Education

PREPARING PHYSICIANS AND NURSES FOR SRMC

SRMC depends on a coordinated administrative, management, clinical, and support program under the direction of a responsible administrator. An informed and progressive medical staff working collaboratively with nursing and support staffs to ensure development, implementation, and maintenance of the highest quality patient care programs is also key to operational success.

It is essential to have a strong physician champion serve as clinical program director. The clinical director assists the SRMC administrator with program development and is responsible for the service's clinical operation. Ideally, the clinical director should be responsible for all the SRMC's clinical services, whether provided by obstetricians, family physicians, pediatricians, anesthesiologists, nurses, midwives, or ancillary personnel. Although this may be difficult to achieve in an organization that already fragments maternity care into separate components of care provided by people reporting to different departments, it is still an important goal that must eventually be achieved to provide optimal consistency and continuity of care.

SRMC Champions

In addition to this physician leader, it is important to identify and develop physician and nurs-

ing champions. Developing a leadership core is a carefully structured and implemented process that is described in Chapter 8. These champions should be opinion leaders who have the respect of their peers. They should include representatives from all the maternity care specialties: obstetrics, pediatrics, neonatology, perinatology, anesthesiology, radiology, and family practice. A respected colleague will best be able to foster change among his or her peers (Lomas, Enkin, Anderson, Hannah, Vayda & Singer, 1991).

Philosophical Understanding

To successfully make changes, the medical and nursing staff must understand and embrace family-centered care principles. A continuing education program, which focuses on SRMC practices, helps physicians and nurses develop knowledge and skills related to providing family-centered care. Physicians respond most positively when taught by other physicians. Usually, outside speakers who have already practiced in family-centered maternity programs can best convince medical staff of SRMC's value in improving quality of care and in benefiting the physicians themselves. Conducted by practicing physicians, the typical presentation begins with a definition and overview of family-centered maternity care followed by a comparison of traditional and family-centered models of care. The physician presenter then describes what must be done to make a successful transition to SRMC. The rest of the time is spent detailing specific clinical strategies incorporating the principles of SRMC into obstetric, pediatric, and neonatal practice. In the course of the discussion, the presenter identifies and responds to participant concerns.

Physician education emphasizes the importance of educating families from preconception through the early years of parenting and of providing this education in their offices, during rounds, and whenever they come into contact with childbearing families. To move from their traditional practices, physicians must be helped to understand the benefits of SRMC for their practices and for the quality of family care. Because program development and implementation can be lengthy, interest can fade. Physicians must be encouraged to stay with the process through frequent, clear, and concise communications from SRMC staff.

Core Competencies for Practice in SRMC Programs

It cannot be assumed that physicians and nurses with sufficient knowledge and skills to practice in obstetrics will necessarily be competent to practice in SRMC programs. Today's healthcare professionals have received little education about normalcy-oriented labor and birth management in either their didactic or clinical education. The attitudes and skills necessary for keeping the birth process physiologic or normal have not been taught along with the skills to perform medical and nursing tasks and procedures.

Competency refers to a minimum standard that protects society, whereas proficiency implies expertise (Benner, 1984). Competency involves integrating performance objectives that reflect cognitive awareness, psychomotor skills, and attitudes (Simpson & Creehan, 1998). A specific set of competencies describes professional practice in an SRMC program. Because collaborative practice is a cornerstone of SRMC, the competencies are the same for physicians and for nurses, even though the specific practices of nursing and medicine require a different focus and emphasis.

In addition to meeting high standards for clinical practice, all medical and nursing staff members who practice in SRMC programs must comply with a set of core competencies that support the SRMC goals. Specifically, these competencies require staff to:

- Establish and participate in providing educational programs designed to inform expectant mothers and their families about the events of the childbearing year.
- Support and encourage the increased participation of women and their families in all appropriate decision-making aspects by providing them with information about medical surveillance and intervention choices.
- Promote and facilitate the provision of family-centered maternity care by encouraging flexibility in attitudes, policies, and procedures.
- Support collaboration among family physicians, certified nurse midwives, obstetrician/gynecologists, pediatricians, select subspecialists (neonatologists, perinatologists, and others), and nurses in providing all aspects of obstetric care.
- Participate in efforts to improve the linkages and coordination among agencies providing maternal–infant antepartum, intrapartum, and postpartum care, with the goal of improving access to care, quality of care, education, and follow-up care for women and infants. Such agencies could include public health organizations, community groups, private physicians, and others.
- Support professional agencies in their attempts to offer continuing medical and nursing education that maintains personnel's competence in providing family-centered maternity care in every community.
- Support the development of curricula to teach physicians and nurses the goals and principles of socially responsive, family-centered maternity care.

Competency Assessment

To determine what education might be needed, SRMC staff development programs begin by assessing current levels of competence so educators understand any deficiencies in skill or knowledge. It is often useful to require that physicians and nurses complete a self-assessment process to measure knowledge and skills in order to identify learning needs. Because the hospital accreditation process requires the organization to assess each staff member's ability to meet performance standards, developing competency assessments for nurses undergoing the change to SRMC may also help the hospital meet JCAHO standards.

The Educational Program

Implementing SRMC programs requires the implementation of a formal educational program that goes beyond achieving clinical competencies. All clinical staff must practice in keeping with the SRMC program's goals and must be competent to provide SRMC. This requires all physicians and nurses to develop a broad range of knowledge, skills, and critical-thinking abilities.

Neither medical nor nursing staff development will be easy or inexpensive in terms of time or resources. However, the payback will come in reduced staff costs, improved quality of care, and increased patient satisfaction (Nathanson, 1985; Olson & Smith, 1992; Reed & Schmid, 1986; *NAWHP Focus,* 1990).

For both physicians and nurses, the use of staff preceptors and mentors can facilitate clinical learning. The number of preceptors selected should equal the number of learners who will be engaged in the process at any given time, so that each preceptor will be responsible for guiding one learner at any given time. Whereas physicians may benefit from spending a single day with a mentor or preceptor, nurses may require the assistance of a preceptor throughout their education period.

Medical Staff Education

To prepare for practice in SRMC programs, physicians complete a continuing medical education (CME) program and certification process that emphasizes provision of family-centered maternity care, including normalcy-oriented labor and birth management and family development. Before and after attendance at this course, each physician attendee completes an SRMC Practice Self-Assessment Scorecard designed to measure knowledge and skills specific to the practice of socially responsible maternity care. This self-assessment serves to guide each physician's learning experiences throughout the course and provide feedback to each participant after completion of the course.

The educational program includes a review of current literature, comparison of their typical practices with those of benchmark SRMC programs, and discussion with colleagues practicing in contemporary SRMC settings. Experts who practice in SRMC programs present lectures. Each workshop participant must complete pretests and posttests for each session to receive the certificate of completion.

After successful completion of this course, participants receive a certificate to indicate their readiness to practice in an SRMC program.

Nursing Staff Preparation

SRMC relies on multiskilled nurses working as a single maternity nursing staff. Nursing care in this model requires an advanced level of clinical and management skills with decreased emphasis on the performance of tasks. Figure 4-1 depicts an SRMC nurse interacting with a mother–baby couple for whom she is providing care.

Transforming conventional maternity nursing practice to SRMC nursing practice requires merging staffs from labor and delivery, postpartum, and well-baby nursery. All nurses working in SRMC programs must be educationally and experientially prepared to care for women and their infants through all stages of the childbirth experience. This requires that most nurses receive additional education. When nurses are multiskilled, fewer nurses may be needed to provide the same services to families on a more comprehensive basis. However, the long-term benefits of increased efficiency and improved productivity will require an investment in staff development. There is no quick fix. Without this investment of time and resources, the educational program will not succeed.

The RN is the primary caregiver and functions as a liaison to other caregivers. The emphasis of nursing practice in SRMC programs is on patient education, family involvement, informed decision making, clinical vigilance, and skilled, limited

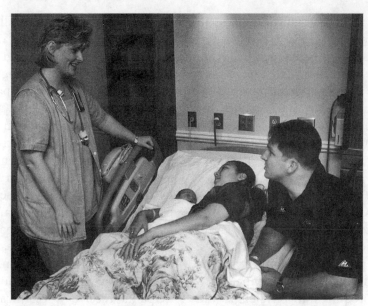

FIGURE 4–1. SRMC nursing requires an advanced level of clinical skills. (Photo courtesy of the Family Maternity Center, Evergreen Hospital Medical Center, Kirkland, WA.)

intervention in the birth and early parenting processes. The SRMC model does not separate mothers from healthy babies. Therefore, newborn admission to the hospital takes place at the mother's bedside. This means that, optimally, each mother–newborn pair has a nurse assigned to their care for the first hour or two after birth. This nursing-care model results in increased use of the knowledge base and strengths of the nurse, greater intellectual challenge, and more professional accountability. This, in turn, results in improved job satisfaction, which is reflected in less staff turnover and decreased absenteeism (Crompton, Maisenbacher, York Eppley & Phillips, 1999; McCloskey, 1988; Schmid & Gerlach, 1986).

The Educational Program

For nurses, the educational program includes maternity theory and skills, critical thinking, change management, service excellence, team building, and communication in the workplace. Nurses also need education in delegation and leadership to collaborate effectively with other team members, including nonlicensed assistive

personnel (Krapohl & Larson, 1996). The initial SRMC educational program is followed by ongoing staff development for staff to maintain and advance in knowledge and skills.

Length of the Educational Program

The amount of time that staff development takes will vary according to staff expertise, previous preparation, and the rates at which different individuals learn. Staff members being educated need to work full time during the clinical orientation regardless of whether they normally do so. During clinical education, nurses are treated like new orientees and are not counted in daily staffing of the maternity program. The educational process concludes when the learner demonstrates the ability to function competently in the new role.

Content of the Educational Program

To ensure success, SRMC programs rely on the assistance of qualified professional educators to plan and conduct educational programs. The program planner develops specific goals and objectives to describe the performance that will be expected of each staff member. Individualized assessments will reveal information about each nurse's strengths and educational needs. The educational program combines didactic and clinical experience, skills labs, mentoring, opportunities for clinical practice, skills review, and competency validation.

Learning new skills can be extremely stressful for staff. It asks confident, experienced, and skilled nurses to return to a state in which they are none of these things. Preceptors, mentors, and instructors must be prepared to help staff cope with their feelings, which may include grief over the temporary loss of their "expert" role, frustration, insecurity, and fear. Educators, preceptors, and mentors can help the learners maintain their sense of humor, focus on their daily progress, and constantly reinforce that they are gaining new knowledge and skills.

Competency Evaluation

To validate competency, the program must set clear goals and performance objectives. Each nurse must demonstrate meeting those objectives before education in SRMC is considered complete. Thereafter, an ongoing evaluation, including an annual written performance evaluation, is required for accreditation.

Practicing in SRMC Programs

It takes collaboration to fulfill the promises of family-centered maternity care. To achieve a successful SRMC program, specialty and subspecialty providers must share strong collegial relationships. Provider and nursing staffs must work in an atmosphere of mutual respect that will facilitate their collaboration in all aspects of providing care for families.

Collaborative Practice

Collaborative practice in maternity care combines the knowledge and skills of the physician provider with those of nonphysician providers, maximizing the efficiency of both the clinicians and the healthcare system (American College of Obstetricians and Gynecologists [ACOG], 1994).

In successful SRMC programs, specialty and subspecialty providers share strong collegial relationships. Obstetricians, family practitioners, and certified nurse-midwives working together in an atmosphere of mutual respect can provide obstetric care for families throughout pregnancy, childbirth, and the postpartum period. Obstetricians, family practitioners, and/or advanced practice nurses such as neonatal or pediatric nurse practitioners can provide infant care.

There are advantages to implementing a model of collaborative practice in SRMC programs to combine the physician provider's knowledge skills with those of nonphysician providers. This model can maximize the efficiency of both the clinicians and the healthcare system (ACOG, 1994).

Definition

The Executive Board of ACOG (ACOG, 1994) has approved the following definition of collaborative practice:

> Collaborative practice in the healthcare of women is a comprehensive, dynamic system of patient-centered healthcare delivered by a multidisciplinary team. The team consists of obstetrician/gynecologists and other healthcare professionals who function within their educational preparation and scope of practice. These team members work together using mutually agreed upon guidelines and policies that define the individual and shared responsibilities of each member.

Nonphysician providers, such as nurse practitioners (NPs), physician assistants (PAs), certified registered nurse anesthetists (CRNAs), and certified nurse-midwives (CNMs) have demonstrated their value and benefits to patients, providers, and the medical practice (ACOG, 1994). NPs, CRNAs, and CNMs are registered nurses with specialty education in primary or acute care, licensed to practice at an advanced level. In collaborative practice, advanced practice nurses, physicians' assistants, and physicians share authority for providing care within the scope of their practice (Wilber, 1997). Midwife-obstetrician collaborative practice offers, perhaps, the best strategy for achieving optimal maternal outcomes (Mvula &

Miller, 1998). CRNAs administer anesthesia and monitor patients during surgeries and during labor, and birth epidurals while under the supervision of physician anesthesiologists.

Although the responsibilities of physicians place them in the role of ultimate authority because of their specialty education and clinical preparation, each team member must communicate well and must trust and respect the others (Stapleton, 1998). The concept of a team guided by one of its own members and the acceptance of shared responsibility for outcomes promotes shared accountability (ACOG, 1994; Sheer, 1996). The biggest winner in collaborative practice is the expectant mother who receives the comprehensive care that a team can provide (Stapleton, 1998).

Nurse-Midwifery

Studies of nurse-midwifery care outcomes reported over the past 70 years document many benefits in both low- and high-risk populations. Examples of these benefits include low rates of cesarean birth and preterm birth, fewer low or very low birth weight babies, less use of oxytocin, fewer episiotomies, fewer severe lacerations, and lower instrumental delivery rates. Further, nurse-midwives incur fewer legal incidents and boast excellent maternal and neonatal outcomes (Goer, 1999; Rooks, 1997). The advantages of quality midwifery care are further enhanced by its cost benefits (Butler, Abrams, Parker, Roberts & Laros, 1993; Clarke, Taffel & Martin, 1997; Ernst, 1996; Rosenblatt, Dobie, Hart, Schneeweiss, Gould, Raine, Benedetti, Pirani & Perrin, 1997). Women also report increased satisfaction with their care. They describe a relationship built on respect, trust, and alliance (Kennedy, 1995). Women who use midwives often experience more personalized care that is more sensitive to their needs and desires (Health Care Advisory Board, 1995). Indeed, midwifery care embodies the values of SRMC.

Because of these many advantages, nurse-midwives working in consultation with obstetricians are an increasingly popular option among both consumers and hospitals. Many hospitals have established midwifery programs (Health

Care Advisory Board, 1995). In some instances, these have been restricted to low-income patients (Blanchette, 1995). In contracting with payers, hospitals typically convey the cost-effectiveness and the continuum of care provided by such midwifery programs.

Nurse-Midwifery and Physician Partnerships

In some SRMC programs, obstetricians practice collaboratively with nurse-midwives. This arrangement can result in lower intervention rates, superior perinatal and maternal care, and improved maternal satisfaction. In addition, these practices demonstrate increased efficiency in obstetric care provision and improved financial profiles for the provider practice (Brown & Grimes, 1995; King & Shah, 1998; Walker & Stone, 1996). Collaborative practice allows each professional to do what he or she does best. Midwives can lower the obstetricians' normal obstetric caseloads, leaving them free to treat complicated or high-risk maternal cases and to perform surgery. Having female midwives available in practices where physician providers are male also provides women with access to a female provider if they wish. This is an especially attractive option to some women.

The decision to form a collaborative practice is influenced by the setting (academic, acute care, ambulatory, managed care, and so forth), community needs, and the number and type of providers in the current practices (ACOG, 1994). In areas that have no shortage of obstetricians, obstetricians may be reluctant to develop collaborative practices for fear of competition. This reluctance is shortsighted as evidenced by a study conducted for the American College of Nurse-Midwives (ACNM) in 1993. The ACNM found that two thirds of the 500 women surveyed would only consider a nurse-midwife if they could have periodic checks during pregnancy from an obstetrician (Braus, 1997). This survey, as well as our experience nationwide, suggests that US women are not looking to replace obstetricians with midwives, but that they would consider an obstetrician-midwife collaborative practice.

As market forces make it imperative to focus on performance, outcome, and especially cost-effectiveness in the delivery of healthcare, collaborative practice becomes more attractive (Dower & O'Neil, 1997). NPs and CNMs can support physician-practice expansion and provide additional choices for women, while lowering the cost of maternity care.

Family Practice

As with advanced practice nurses, the issue of family practice is often influenced by the setting, community needs, and the number and type of providers available in the community. Although the majority of family physicians do not deliver babies (Larimore & Reynolds, 1994), there is evidence that family physicians can reduce many obstetric interventions while maintaining good maternal and neonatal outcomes (Deutchman, Connor & Sills, 1995; Goer, 1999; Hart, Rosenblatt, Fordyce, Pirani, Baldin & Dobie, 1996; Jasper and Jordan, 1995; Larimore & Reynolds, 1994). Consumer research reveals that many women like the idea of a family practice physician for maternity and child care because it offers continuity of care for mother and child (Larimore & Reynolds, 1994).

Staff for Community Educational Programs

Often, organizations assign childbirth educational programming to a staff person with other maternity unit responsibilities. Employing a full-time childbirth educational program manager ensures comprehensive program development as well as a champion for educational services for families in the family-centered environment. This helps to ensure the educational program's success. Without a program manager's leadership, even when the program offers a range of classes, they remain just that—classes, rather than one element of a programmatic approach to education. They will contribute little to the organization's overall success in achieving the goals of SRMC. In addition, the satisfaction levels of the mother and her family with the program can be low and attendance poor.

The childbirth educational program's manager has primary responsibility for program design, staff hiring, supervision and development of childbirth educators, oversight of the registration procedure, integration of the educational program with other professional and clinical services, ongoing program evaluation, and community networking. Frequently, this manager also has responsibilities for teaching various classes as well as for managing lactation services and other perinatal programs offered by the organization, such as those related to bereavement support for parents.

Program Registrar

The program registrar facilitates easy access to the childbirth educational program for women and their families. Parents frequently remember the registrar by name, showing the significance of the first contact that parents have with an organization. The majority of childbirth educational program registration can be done by mail, and parents appreciate this streamlined approach that reduces the need to connect by phone. The registrar, however, plays a central role in helping parents who have complicated needs either in terms of schedules or pregnancy experiences.

Successful childbirth educational programs make every effort to enroll each parent into their desired class or other acceptable program. Rule-driven organizations often remind parents that no classes are available when they register late. Family-centered organizations search for solutions with the family. The value of this both in terms of public relations and health outcomes cannot be overestimated. Families who seek service at the last moment often have complicated lives or pregnancy experiences. These families benefit greatly from educational services designed for health promotion.

Clerical Support

Clerical support expedites the work of the educators and the program coordinator. The program clerical staff member is responsible for room scheduling and classroom setup, maintaining adequate supplies of class materials, and other secretarial duties. In smaller programs, one person performs all duties for both the registration and clerical positions.

Educator Staff

Childbirth educators are of critical importance to the childbirth program's success. The childbirth educator often spends more time with the expectant family than any other professional—an average of 12 hours. SRMC programs require all childbirth educators to complete a nationally recognized certification program. We recommend a certification program that includes self-study, observation of a complete class series, labor observation, student teaching for a complete series, and an examination process. Somewhat abbreviated programs are available for staff who already have extensive teaching experience.

The childbirth educational program may employ a wide range of educators, for example, lactation counselors, infant massage specialists, postnatal educators, and grief counselors. Certification programs in many of these and other areas are available and may supplement or replace the childbirth educator certification requirement based on the organization's needs. Regardless of his or her background, it is critical that the educator has both skill and knowledge in adult education principles. Ongoing staff development achieved through both in-house programs and attendance at national conferences is essential for maintaining a quality educational service.

Clinical Practice Parameters in SRMC Programs

In healthcare today, the focus on quality and accountability continues to intensify with purchasers and consumers looking for best value when buying health coverage. The importance of using evidence to guide health practice and decisions about medical necessity is being stressed.

Evidence-Based Practice

Evidence published by professional organizations and professional training and educational programs all contribute to establishing the body of knowledge on which SRMC providers base their practice. "Evidence-based" care means incorporating into practice a well-analyzed combination of professional expertise and information from reliable sources that has been systematically gathered and thoroughly reviewed (Association of Women's Health, Obstetric and Neonatal Nurses, 1998). To assist physicians in developing competencies for providing normalcy-oriented labor and birth care, SRMC programs use the best available current evidence to evaluate maternity care practices.

Perhaps the foremost source of data for evidence-based care is the Cochrane Database of Systematic Reviews (CDSR). The Cochrane Database is an ongoing series of meta-analyses of randomized clinical trials supplemented with findings of studies conducted by other methods. The database, titled the "Oxford Database of Perinatal Trials," is available on compact disk and is updated quarterly. *A Guide to Effective Care in Pregnancy and Childbirth* contains the conclusions of these analyses (Enkin, Keirse, Renfrew & Neilson, 1995). Appendices identify forms of care that (1) are clearly beneficial, (2) are likely to prove beneficial, (3) have tradeoffs between benefits and adverse effects, (4) are of unknown effectiveness, (5) are unlikely to prove beneficial, and (6) are likely to be ineffective or harmful. The large body of scientific data summarized in the Cochrane Database forms the basis of physiologic childbirth management, prenatal education, and enhanced social and psychological support from caregivers during the childbearing experience.

Cesarean Change Strategies

Evaluating cesarean sections for appropriateness is an ongoing challenge for hospitals and medical staffs. We have found that cesarean section rates are a logical place to begin working to lower obstetric average length of stay (ALOS) and to improve the quality of care for families because so much variation occurs in these rates. The US total cesarean birth rate has decreased in recent years from a high point of 25% in 1988 to 21.8% in 1996. Since the mid-1980s, however, almost one million cesareans have been performed each year in the United States (Flamm, Berwick & Kabcenell, 1998). The lowest cesarean delivery rates continue to be in the West and the highest rates in the South (*Monthly Vital Statistical Report,* 1998).

In 1990, the Department of Health and Human Services set a Healthy People 2000 goal of reducing the cesarean rate to 15% by the year 2000 (Rooks, 1997). National cesarean rates of many countries, including the United Kingdom, Denmark, and Sweden, are less than 15% while maintaining lower infant mortality rates than the United States.

Strategies to decrease the variation in cesarean birth rates have been widely published in the literature (Sanchez-Ramos et al., 1990; Schimmel et al., 1997). For physicians, CME programs on interaction between physician practice parameters, length of stay, and costs is a good place to start. Controlling practice patterns such as elective inductions, admission of patients in false or very early labor, and early labor epidurals can be effective in reducing the rate as can simply allowing more labor time. Physiologic labor positioning as well as one-to-one support throughout labor by a professional birth attendant, nurse, certified nurse-midwife, or doula can help women manage pain and tolerate labor (Hodnett, 1995; Flamm, Berwick & Kabcenell, 1998). Although there has been recent controversy regarding vaginal birth after cesarean (VBAC) (Sachs & Castro, 1999), it remains true that VBAC is a safe, effective means of giving birth for women with one prior, transverse uterine scar. Thus, it remains a safe, effective means of reducing the cesarean rate according to the best available evidence (ACOG, 1998).

Practice Parameters

Practice parameters are strategies for managing care, developed to assist clinical decision making. Practice parameters define appropriate care and help standardize the indications for procedures (Meeker, 1992). They are important to ensure that clinical staff members perform procedures appropriately, and they reduce the number of procedures done for marginal indications. Well-designed parameters allow for local variables and are sufficiently flexible to permit the exercise of medical judgment and individualizing care.

Establishing practice parameter targets involves a collaborative planning process among management, providers, and hospital administrators. Potential outcomes suitable for setting targets include ALOS, cesarean delivery rate, VBAC, labor induction rates, epidural use, non-birth-related antepartum admission and discharge rates, use of outpatient services, and others.

Guidelines

Guidelines lay out generally accepted approaches to care. As with practice parameters, there is leeway for medical judgment and individualizing care (Meeker, 1992). Research evidence and expert opinion form the basis for guidelines that are developed by the professional associations whose members provide care for childbearing families.

Care Pathways

A care pathway is a road map of the patient-care process. It sequences the important tasks that patients need and describes who should perform them. It allows care to be given in a predictable and timely way. Care pathways help to achieve desired patient outcomes with appropriate lengths of stay. They do not replace physician orders or nursing standards of care, but are plans for patient care that contain essential elements of care that may be considered. Care pathways can also help providers control costs by identifying and preventing adverse situations that may prolong hospitalization.

Hospitals develop coordinated care pathways for maternal and newborn patients that describe care during the childbearing year. Coordinating this care requires a multidisciplinary effort involving management, nursing staff, physicians, and other providers involved in the family's care. During the process of pathway development, physicians clarify their standing orders for everyone involved, including the woman and her family. Women receive copies of all care pathways at the beginning of their prenatal care. At each visit, women and their healthcare providers can discuss progress along the pathway, and women can be encouraged to give their input to its development. During hospitalization, nurses keep the pathway at the bedside so both the new mother and nurses can refer to it daily. This detailed account of what the woman can expect for herself and her infant helps the mother work with her providers and nursing staff toward mutually planned goals (Driscoll & Caico, 1996).

Standards

Unlike guidelines and practice parameters, standards require justification for deviations. This makes them the most appropriate tools for evaluating care. Standards apply only to those aspects of care for which there is consensus (Meeker, 1992). In SRMC programs, clinicians evaluate compliance with standards of practice and important clinical outcomes.

QUALITY MANAGEMENT

In successful programs, providers collaborate with the organization's administration to commit to a practice philosophy that maternity care services can always improve, and they have an ongoing commitment to that improvement. As part of that commitment, SRMC quality management programs rely on the use of process and outcome indicators to measure improvements in the quality of patient care as well as operational efficiency of the program as a whole.

Process management allows the organization and its providers to respond quickly to concerns about the quality of care as such concerns arise, regardless of who raises the concern. Outcomes management uses measurement tools to monitor, evaluate, and improve clinical outcomes while better using resources (Flarey, 1995). The focus is on developing a normalcy-based approach to patient care within a framework of concern about developing cost-effective systems and strategies. The process of peer review becomes educational rather than punitive.

Another part of the commitment is maintaining an ongoing quality improvement program that promotes professional education and research and includes periodic evaluations of staff and services. Many successful SRMC programs develop report cards to inform consumers about results of the organization's quality management program so they are informed consumers of services offered in the SRMC program. Because provider practice is one important area that is monitored as part of the organization's overall focus on quality improvement, report cards often report provider intervention rates and practice data for individual physicians and for the organization as a whole. (See Chapter 8.)

The SRMC program's physician quality improvement plan measures adherence to the goals of SRMC and to clinical practice standards. Specific indicators are designed to measure the quality of clinical care, patient satisfaction, and unit financial performance. Regularly published reports communicate analysis results to consumers and to the medical community. In successful SRMC programs, management, providers, and nurses work together to achieve the SRMC program's desired outcomes.

SUMMARY

In SRMC programs, providers are viewed as valued stakeholders. Gaining physician loyalty will not be sufficient to guarantee the development of an exemplary clinical product. A successful program grows from collaborative relationships among management, physicians, and nonphysician providers. It requires physician involvement in overall planning and evaluation, and it especially requires understanding and practice of mother–baby nursing and physiologic labor and birth management. SRMC relies on a multiskilled nursing staff educated to care for women and their infants through all stages of the childbirth experience. Wise program planners motivate and guide physicians and nurses through what may be a stressful and time-consuming process.

REFERENCES

American College of Obstetricians and Gynecologists. (1994). *Guidelines for implementing collaborative practice*. Washington, DC: Author.

American College of Obstetricians and Gynecologists. (1998). *ACOG practice bulletin*. ACOG #2 VBAC. Washington, D.C.: Author.

Association of Women's Health, Obstetric and Neonatal Nurses. (1998). *Standards and guidelines for professional nursing practice in the care of women and newborns* (5th ed.). Washington, DC: Author.

Benner, P. (1984). *From novice to expert*. Menlo Park, CA: Addison-Wesley.

Blanchette, H. (1995). Comparison of obstetric outcome of a primary-care access clinic staffed by certified nurse-midwives and a private practice group of obstetricians in the same community. *American Journal of Obstetrics and Gynecology, 172*(6), 1864–1868.

Braus, P. (1997). *Marketing health care to women*. Ithaca, NY: American Demographics Books.

Brown, S. A., & Grimes, D. E. (1995, November/December). A meta-analysis of nurse midwives and nurse practitioners in primary care. *Nursing Research, 44*(6), 332–339.

Butler, J., Abrams, B., Parker, J., Roberts, J. M., and Laros, R. K., Jr. (1993). Supportive nurse-midwife care is associated with a reduced incidence of cesarean section. *American Journal of Obstetrics and Gynecology, 168*, 1407–1413.

Clarke, S. C., Taffel, S. M., & Martin, J. A. (1997). Trends and characteristics of births attended by midwives. *Statistical Bulletin of the Metropolitan Insurance Company, 78*(1), 9–18.

Crompton, D. A., Maisenbacher Roth, R., York Eppley, G., & Phillips, C. R. (1999). Follow family-focused care principles. *Nursing Management, 30*(2), 47–50.

Deutchman, M. E., Connor, P. D., & Sills, D. (1995). Perinatal outcomes: A comparison between family physicians and obstetricians. *Journal of the American Board of Family Practice, 8*(6), 440–447.

Dower, C., & O'Neil, E. (1997). Collaborative practice, regulation, and market forces: A changing health care agenda. *Women's Health Issues, 7*(5), 298–300.

Driscoll, D., & Caico, C. (1996). Critical pathways and mother–baby coupling. *Nursing Management, 27*(12), 22–25.

Enkin, M., Keirse, M. J. N. C., Renfrew, M., & Neilson, J. (1995). *A guide to effective care in pregnancy and childbirth* (2nd ed.). Oxford: Oxford University Press.

Ernst, K. M. (1996). Midwifery, birth centers, and healthcare reform. *Journal of Obstetric, Gynecologic, and Neonatal Nursing, 25*, 433–439.

Flamm, B. L., Berwick, D. M., & Kabcenell, A. (1998). Reducing cesarean section rates safely: Lessons from a "Breakthrough Series" collaborative. *Birth, 25*(2), 117–124.

Flarey, D. L. (1995). *Redesigning nursing care delivery: Transforming our future*. Philadelphia, PA: J. B. Lippincott.

Goer, H. (1999). *The thinking woman's guide to a better birth*. New York, NY: Perigee.

Hart, L. G., Rosenblatt, R. A., Fordyce, M., Pirani, M. J., Baldin, L. M., & Dobie, S. A. (1996). Rural and urban differences in physician resource use for low-risk obstetrics. *Health Services Research, 31*(4), 429–452.

Health Care Advisory Board. (1995, July). *Project #3: Hospital-based midwifery programs*. Washington, DC: Author.

Hodnett, E. D. (1995). Support from caregivers during childbirth. (Computer software.) In: M. J. N. C. Keirse, M. J. Renfrew, J. P. Neilson & C. Crowther (Eds.), *Cochrane database of systematic reviews* (disk issue 2). London: BMJ Publishing Group.

Jasper, D., & Jordan, J. (1995). Family medicine in a tertiary care hospital. Obstetrical outcomes and interventions. *Canadian Family Physician, 41*, 601–607.

Kennedy, H. P. (1995). The essence of nurse-midwifery care: The woman's story. *Journal of Nurse-Midwifery, 40*(5), 410–417.

King, T., & Shah, M. A. (1998, January/February). Integrated midwife physician practice. *Journal of Nurse Midwifery, 43*(1), 55–60.

Krapohl, G. L., & Larson, E. (1996). The impact of unlicensed assistive personnel on nursing care delivery. *Nursing Economic\$, 14*(2), 99–110.

Larimore, W. L., & Reynolds, J. L. (1994). Family practice maternity care in America: Ruminations on reproducing an endangered species—Family physicians who deliver babies. *Journal of the American Board of Family Practice, 7*(6), 478–488.

Lomas, J., Enkin, M. W., Anderson, G., Hannah, W., Vayda, E., & Singer, J. (1991). Opinion leaders vs. audit and feedback to implement practice guidelines: Delivery after previous cesarean section. *Journal of the American Medical Association, 265*, 2202–2207.

McCloskey, S. (1988). *Job satisfaction comparisons between nurses working in mother–baby units and nurses cross-trained in labor and delivery, postpartum, and nursery*. Unpublished master's thesis, University of Akron, Akron, OH.

Meeker, C. I. (1992). A consensus-based approach to practice parameters. *Obstetrics and Gynecology, 79*(5), 790–793.

Mvula, M. M., & Miller, J. M., Jr. (1998). A comparative evaluation of collaborative prenatal care. *Obstetrics and Gynecology, 91*(2), 169–173.

Nathanson, M. (1985, March 29). Single-room maternity care seen as way to attract patients, cut costs. *Modern Healthcare, 15*(7), 72, 74.

National Center for Health Statistics (1998). *Monthly Vital Statistical Report, 46*(11S), 17–18.

Olson, M. E., & Smith, M. J. (1992). An evaluation of single-room maternity care. *Health Care Supervisor, 11*(1), 43–49.

Reed, G., & Schmid, M. (1986, September/October). Nursing implementation of single-room maternity care. *Journal of Obstetric, Gynecologic, and Neonatal Nursing, 15,* 386–389.

Rooks, J. P. (1997). *Midwifery and childbirth in America.* Philadelphia: Temple University Press.

Rosenblatt, R. A., Dobie, S. A., Hart, L. G., Schneeweiss, R., Gould, D., Raine, T. R., Benedetti, T. J., Pirani, M. J., & Perrin, E. B. (1997). Interspecialty differences in the obstetric care of low-risk women. *American Journal of Public Health, 87,* 344–351.

Sachs, B. P., & Castro, M. A. (1999). The risks of lowering the cesarean-delivery rate. *New England Journal of Medicine, 340*(1), 54–57.

Sanchez-Ramos, L., Kaunitz, A. M., Peterson, H. B., Martinez-Schnell, B., & Thompson, R. J. (1990). Reducing cesarean sections at a teaching hospital. *American Journal of Obstetrics and Gynecology, 163*(3), 1081–1087.

Schimmel, L. M., DeJoseph, J., & Schimmel, L. D. (1997). Toward lower cesarean birth rates and effective care: Five years' outcomes of joint private obstetric practice. *Birth, 24*(3), 181–187.

Schmid, M., & Gerlach, C. (1986). LDRP: Staffing a single care maternity system. *Nursing Management, 17*(8), 36–40.

Sheer, B. (1996). Reaching collaboration through empowerment: A developmental process. *Journal of Obstetric, Gynecologic, and Neonatal Nursing, 25,* 513–517.

Simpson, K. R., & Creehan, P. A. (1998). *Competence validation for perinatal care providers: Orientation, continuing education and evaluation.* Philadelphia: Lippincott-Raven.

Single-room maternity care brings more patients and higher staff satisfaction. (1990, Spring). *NAWHP Focus,* 7.

Stapleton, S. R. (1998). Team-building: Making collaborative practice work. *Journal of Nurse-Midwifery, 43*(1), 12–18.

Walker, P. H., & Stone, P. W. (1996, Fall). Exploring cost and quality. *Journal of Health Care Finance, 23*(1), 23–47.

Wilber, K. (1997). Collaborative practice and health plans. *Women's Health Issues, 7*(5), 293–297.

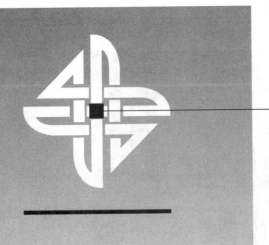

Single-Room Maternity Care Facility Design

Although families find good beginnings in many different environments, both within and outside of medical institutions, a well-designed facility is a key element in achieving the goals of SRMC. A building affects the way that families, staff, and visitors feel about themselves and the service, and can also support the way that they function and interact. A building can communicate the attitudes and priorities of its designers. Even before entering a building, people form judgments about what takes place inside and about the quality of medical care that they will receive (Carpman & Grant, 1993). Figure 5-1 is of Sutter Maternity and Surgery Center, a freestanding 30-bed specialty hospital in Santa Cruz, California.

A maternity facility is also a tool to help the program of care to function. If it is designed from the outset so that every detail supports and facilitates the program goals, the building will not only be comfortable and efficient for client families, visitors, and staff, but will also guide activities in the desired direction. For example, a convenient charting and communications station at the bedside will facilitate decentralization and promote nursing at the patient's bedside. The opposite is also true. Systems designed to accommodate conventional staffing and service patterns, like the multitransfer system and its variant, the labor/delivery/recovery (LDR), will tend to perpetuate conventional clinical care practices.

It is difficult to integrate new approaches to care into existing practice if the facility design does not support these new approaches.

SRMC FACILITY DESIGN

The SRMC facility is a fresh approach to maternity design. The SRMC facility is an example of socially responsible design as described by Carpman and Grant (1993) in their book, *Design That Cares: Planning Health Care Facilities for Patients and Visitors*. It results from an explicit value system, which in this case is the philosophy and program of single-room maternity care. In a socially responsible design for maternity care, the social, psychological, and physical needs of the woman and her family, of visitors and staff are given first priority. It is developed through a knowledge-based, participatory design process, which includes periodic development of the design and postoccupancy review.

The SRMC facility is designed to meet a number of different needs for each of the groups who will use it, and to help them to work together to achieve a sound family beginning (Figure 5-2). At all times, the medical, emotional, and social needs of the woman and her family must be met through the staff and family collaboration. Some of these needs would be in conflict in a conventional obstetric design. SRMC is a design solution

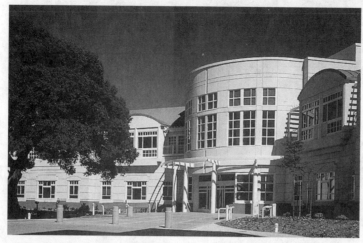

FIGURE 5–1. Sutter Maternity and Surgery Center, Santa Cruz, CA. (Photo courtesy of Sutter Maternity and Surgery Center.)

that meets the family's needs for nonseparation while also meeting a variety of task-related and personal needs of medical, nursing, and other professional staff.

Goals of SRMC Design

The SRMC facility design was developed for the sole purpose of supporting the family-centered goals of the SRMC program of care. These are to provide a program of care that results in:

Healthy mothers and healthy babies. The building facilitates the provision of quality medical and nursing care for the mother and her baby. Depending on the level of care offered by the program, this may include high-acuity services such as a neonatal intensive care nursery or an obstetric intensive-care unit.

Mothers who can successfully parent their babies through the first year of life. The facility supports the mother's learning about newborn care by providing an environment that facilitates a

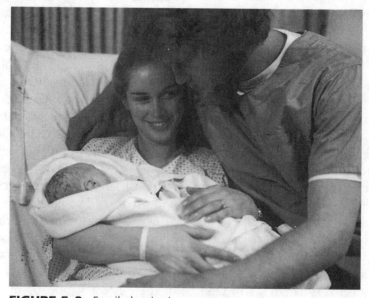

FIGURE 5–2. Family beginning.

normal birthing experience and by providing a comfortable environment that is conducive to education and parent–infant attachment.

Parents who make conception, pregnancy, birth, and childcare choices that are in the best interests of the baby and family. The facility supports family empowerment and development through the provision of space for family participation, education, lactation, support, and counseling.

Families that are confident, nurturing, and enduring. The facility helps the mother and father participate in their family's care by creating an environment that facilitates family participation in care. The design supports family formation by providing a comfortable environment in which the family may remain together without disruption. There are no unnecessary transfers from room to room during important times of the childbearing experience.

Additional goals for the SRMC facility are to provide an environment for:

Cost-effective operation. The facility optimizes operational efficiency through innovative approaches to use of space, staffing, patient flow, material handling, and other aspects of operation. The facility is designed to be built and operated at the least cost that still meets the needs of the SRMC program.

A satisfied and productive staff. Medical, nursing, and other professional staff are provided with facilities that are efficient and pleasant to work in and that meet the needs of quality clinical care. The facility provides not only for task-related activities but also for privacy, relaxation, communication, and education for the people who work there.

An identity as the best place for family beginnings. The design clearly communicates the organization's commitment to giving families the best possible start in life through its location, external appearance, interior design, and provision of resources.

Facility Development Process

The facility development process for SRMC is unlike that of a conventional or evolving clinical service. As with the introduction of other new and specialized services, SRMC requires that the parent organization learn about how SRMC has a different relationship with, requirements of, and contribution to the organization. SRMC has the potential of having an important impact on the attainment of the organization's strategic goals, and its development requires active participation of the organization's leadership and specialized knowledge of the program and its facility requirements. The facility and program development process is integrated under the overall control of the SRMC developer, as illustrated in Figure 5-3.

The SRMC program must be clearly defined in all its important details before starting on facility design or making decisions about facility location. Whether the developer or an independent architect provides the architectural component of strategic planning, the architect's function is to respond to program requirements, as set out by the program developers.

Facility program and space definition is a product of the strategic planning process described in Chapter 6. The project proceeds through functional and space programming that determines the size, scope, and character of the service.

ELEMENTS OF SRMC FACILITY DESIGN

The SRMC facility comprises areas that are arranged to provide for the needs of families, visitors, and staff in an SRMC program of care. The relationship of spaces is similar to that of a hotel, and comparison with the hotel model will illustrate concepts that apply well to the SRMC facility model.

Space Plan

A hotel has public spaces in which initial interaction with guests takes place. Public spaces are welcoming, efficient, and communicate the purpose and style of the institution. Beyond the public spaces, there are specialized, more private lodging and meeting areas where guests are provided the service for which they came. The char-

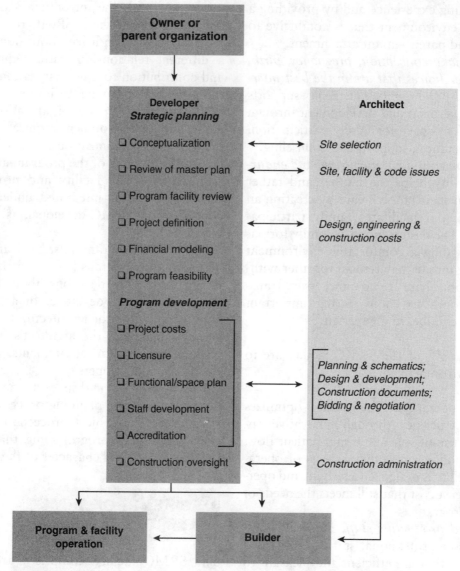

FIGURE 5–3. The recommended SRMC development process integrates facility and design planning and development from strategic planning through completion of the project.

acter of these spaces is in keeping with that of the public areas, but the ambience is in keeping with their function, which is to provide comfort, privacy, and security. The public and guest spaces are unobtrusively supported by a comprehensive and mostly invisible infrastructure that provides food, security, communication, maintenance, housekeeping, business operations, and all other services that enable the hotel to function in a safe, satisfying, and efficient manner.

SRMC facility design reflects a similar arrangement of public, guest (family), service, and staff areas to provide optimal efficiency of operation while preserving a comfortable environment for the family and staff. However, although there is much to be learned from the hospitality industry when it comes to facility design, it must always be clear that the goals of maternity care are more than providing hospitality. Ensuring clinical safety and supporting the important emotional and social transformations that occur around childbirth are expressed in design solutions particular to the SRMC program and facility.

General Layout of Facilities for SRMC

The basic element of the SRMC facility is a cluster of labor/delivery/recovery/postpartum (LDRP) rooms surrounding a central communication/ service core (Fenwick, 1979). This layout allows for the family to remain in the same room, cared for by the same nursing staff on the unit, for the entire maternity stay. Equipment and supplies stored in the central core are taken to the individual LDRP rooms when needed, and are returned to the core for resupply (Fenwick & Dearing, 1981). See Figure 5-4 for a concept drawing of a single cluster with associated cesarean birth rooms and staff areas.

The cluster is supported by spaces for public, family, surgery, babies with needs that cannot be met in the family room, for staff, and for support of facility operations. The separation of spaces provides an appropriate environment for each function, allows for staff and family to work together, and optimizes efficiency of operation. The ratio of these support spaces to the clinical care space is a critical planning concern (Basler, 1981). In SRMC, the LDRP room space is approximately doubled to accommodate public, staff, and support spaces.

A single-cluster SRMC facility will serve a low-volume SRMC program. The size of the cluster is limited by the distance of LDRP rooms from the entrance, control station, equipment storage area, and by other factors. An SRMC service is generally located within a hospital building or a free-standing center, where it is supported by and associated with other services.

Although multiple cluster units can be built into hospital shells, this design works particularly well in a separate building with its own character. (See Figure 5-5 for multiple clusters.) The SRMC

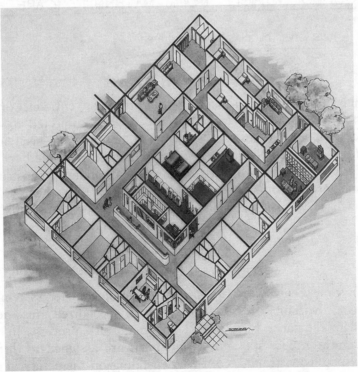

FIGURE 5–4. Original concept drawing of a single cluster with associated cesarean birth rooms.

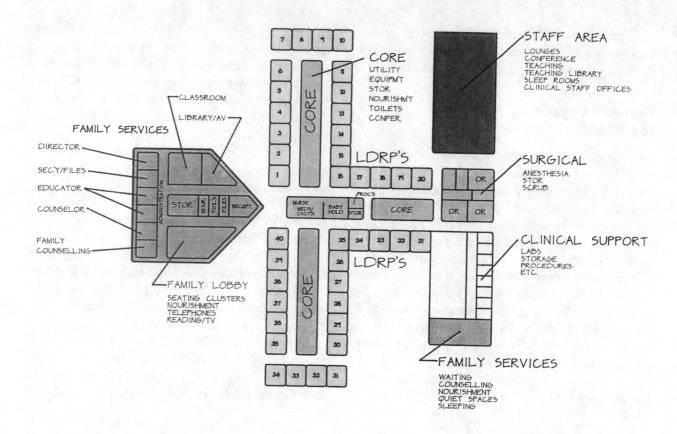

FIGURE 5–5. Multiple clusters served by a common core area.

unit can be a separate, new maternity service in a hospital, or it can be in a women's center where it is associated with women's or ambulatory surgical services. The women's center could either be in a freestanding structure or connected to a hospital by a bridge or tunnel, or the women's center could be part of a specialized women's specialty hospital.

over the conventional or LDR multitransfer model when subjected to mathematical modeling, it has not yet been implemented. Because its relevance is limited to planners considering a major remodel or construction of a large level III or IV facility, the reader is invited to skip to the next section of this chapter if this information is not relevant.

Acuity Gradient

First proposed by Phillips and Fenwick in 1990, the acuity gradient is a variant of SRMC designed to accommodate the large birth volume, wide range of clinical needs, specialized nursing services and space constraints commonly found in large teaching hospitals. Although this concept has significant benefits

Acuity Gradient Space/Program Concept

In the multitransfer system, women are moved through specialized areas according to stages in the maternity process. In the acuity gradient, women are assigned to different LDRP clusters depending on the acuity of nursing care needed. In most cases, the woman will remain in the same room throughout her stay.

The spatial relationship of the maternity care rooms in the acuity gradient is comparable to a piano keyboard. The high-acuity rooms transition to medium-acuity rooms that transition to low-acuity rooms. Within this spectrum of capabilities, groups of rooms are clustered together according to manageable nursing units, proximity to services, environmental considerations, manageability, and available space. The high-acuity rooms are large LDRP rooms specially equipped to handle high-risk obstetric and neonatal care needs.

Each of these rooms is equipped with a full complement of equipment necessary for obstetric intensive care. The high-acuity end of the "keyboard" is separated off as an obstetric intensive-care unit (OBICU) close to the surgical suite, neonatal intensive-care unit (NICU), and other acute-care services. The intermediate portion is the largest section, functioning as a regular SRMC service for most women falling into the normal range of obstetric need. The low-acuity end provides a step-down setting requiring a lesser acuity of nursing care. Figure 5-6 depicts specialized clusters as used in the acuity gradient.

The OBICU

The OBICU is the focal point of high-acuity nursing and subspecialty medical care. Women would be admitted to this end of the acuity gradient according to clinical need, regardless of their stage in the maternity process. For example, the OBICU could serve unstable, high-risk antepartum patients, women at particularly high risk for problems during labor or birth, women whose babies are expected to need immediate resuscitation or intensive care, and also postpartum or postsurgical women who require special attention. A separate OBICU would meet high-risk needs better than a multitransfer unit using LDR rooms does. This is because an LDR room suite typically is used for both high-risk obstetric patients and normal births, and in a large service this would be a busy, noisy environment. This is not appropriate for women receiving intensive care, especially those who have to remain on the unit for many days and for those with fragile medical conditions such as preeclampsia. Because the OBICU is used only for the high-acuity end of the clinical care spectrum, it can be a small, quiet, specialized unit suitably staffed and equipped for intensive care.

The SRMC Birthing Clusters

By removing the high-risk end of the maternity population to an OBICU, the acuity gradient allows the operation of a smaller and less frenetic SRMC unit for the normal-risk birthing population. The LDRP clusters would be more conventionally equipped for childbirth, and specialized equipment would only be brought into the room when needed. This SRMC portion of the acuity gradient could serve the needs of all

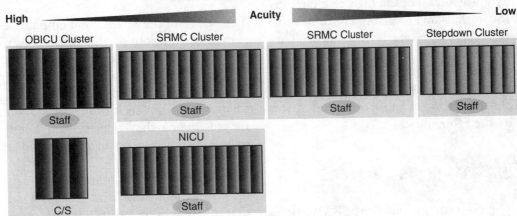

FIGURE 5–6. Specialized clusters as utilized in the Acuity Gradient.

but the highest end of the acuity spectrum, or approximately 80% to 90% of the women birthing on the unit. In addition to providing for labor, delivery, recovery, and postpartum care, the LDRP unit provides an environment for mother–baby nursing.

Step-Down Care

The low-acuity end of the acuity gradient is for use by women who require a low acuity of nursing care. For example, stable postsurgical women, women requiring antenatal hospitalization, and women admitted for clinical workup, could be accommodated in a comfortable, "low-tech" environment that did not have to be adjacent to the bustle of the high-activity components of the acuity gradient. In units with large birth volumes, there could be enough postsurgical women to occupy an entire cluster, particularly in a unit with a high operative delivery rate. A low-acuity cluster would be equipped with comfortable regular beds and optimized for postsurgical mother–baby nursing care. The acuity of nursing and requirement for equipment would be less than in a unit in which babies were born. Where there is limited space for a maternity service in one location, this part of the acuity gradient can be conveniently disconnected from the SRMC unit to create an obstetric step-down unit at some reasonable distance away from the main maternity unit.

Summary of Acuity Gradient

In the acuity gradient, all of the high-risk families are cared for in the same location, concentrating highest skills where they are needed most. This approach also simplifies anesthesia, preparation for surgery, and resuscitation. Except for the small number of admissions to the OBICU, families are able to remain in one room and to be cared for by the same nurses.

SRMC IN WOMEN'S CENTERS

There is a good synergy between SRMC programs and other services in women's maternity/ surgery centers. LDRP rooms can be used flexibly, either for maternity care or for postsurgery recovery. The ambience of a contemporary SRMC service is consistent with the environment desired for other women's services provided in the center, and both services can share most public spaces such as lobby and reception areas, education and resource facilities, business office, access parking, and entrancing. Other program elements such as diagnostic services and surgery support also support the maternity program, thus reducing duplication of expensive facility elements and increasing their utilization.

DESIGN CONSIDERATIONS FOR AN SRMC FACILITY

There are four major flow patterns within the SRMC unit. These patterns apply to families, visitors, staff, and materials.

Flow Patterns

Each flow pattern is considered during the concept design development to ensure clinical safety, efficiency, and the preservation of a comfortable and supportive environment for families and staff. To the extent that it is practical, staff and materials traffic are separated. Descriptive information is then prepared to identify these flow patterns and the interrelationship between patterns and potential points of conflict.

Ambience

The design of the SRMC unit emphasizes the consumer orientation of the facility as well as its functionality and cost-effectiveness. Unlike birthing rooms and alternative birthing centers, the facility does not strive for a residential feeling. "Patients do not seek homeyness any more than they do when they register at a hotel. But they expect comfort, consideration and efficiency" (Carpman & Grant, 1993).

The ambience for maternity care is designed to reflect the mission and beliefs of the service—that birth is a beautiful, transforming, natural event, and that it is a foundation of new family life. Also important is the need for the facility to communicate clinical competence, efficiency, and security. Creating an overall design theme and detailing its implementation are unique to every project. Careful consideration is paid to the customs, attitudes, and beliefs held by the different cultures with which the facility will interact, and design is sensitive to their perceptions and needs.

Colors, contract-quality furniture, and accessories similar to those of a contemporary first-rate hotel are used. Overall, the design promotes the sense that birth is a wellness event with attention shown to the needs and wants of the consumers of the service. The total environment provides a pleasant place for both families and staff.

Light

In creating a warm, relaxed ambience, the use of light is important. Numerous studies have pointed to the importance of light to human behavior. When planners alter light and color, they are exerting an influence on patient and visitor impression (Flynn, 1978). The general room illumination should be diffuse, dimmable, and with good color rendition (Beck, 1984). To achieve a warmly illuminated environment, incandescent lighting is preferred. Windows in

each patient care room and in staff areas are essential to provide natural light for physical and mental health. The purest and best light is sunlight, and it remains a major reference standard for assessing light quality (Sisson, 1978). Open spaces, high ceilings, skylights, and well-lit areas help to communicate a welcoming, reassuring environment (Figure 5-7). It is important that families have control over their environment's lighting, including window shading and the intensity of illumination.

Noise

The typical noise of health care facilities is a source of stress for many hospital patients and visitors (Hurst, 1966). In an SRMC unit, particular attention is paid to control of sound arising from nursing, housekeeping activities, and patients, visitors, and activities in the LDRP rooms. Noise control begins with the initial siting of the functional areas of the unit, and continues with facility layout, architectural and interior design, in-wall and door insulation, wall and floor coverings, and acoustic screening. LDRP room doors should be sound insulated, and families should be able to control whether the doors are open or closed. These measures, together with avoidance of loud talking and care in handling

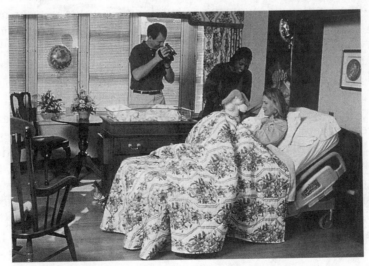

FIGURE 5–7. In creating a warm, relaxed ambience, the use of light is important. (Photo courtesy of Wellstar Family Birthplace, Cobb Hospital, Austell, GA.)

equipment, are effective approaches to noise control (Carpman & Grant, 1993).

Communications

Communication capabilities are provided between clinical staff, between medical staff, patients and visitors, and between all groups and the outside world. To promote collaborative practice in the SRMC facility, the facility is wired for telephone, intercom, computer, and radio communication capabilities and is designed to easily accept future technologies. A synchronized clock system is a high priority in the SRMC unit because of medical/legal issues related to timing.

DESIGN CONSIDERATIONS FOR PUBLIC AREAS

The influence of the facility's design begins with the public's first view of the structure in its surroundings.

Location and Wayfinding

If the SRMC unit is in a new specialty women's hospital, the buildings and surrounding environment can be optimized for functional efficiency, for family and staff comfort, and to communicate the quality and philosophy of the services provided. Generally, maternity and women's services will share a common parking, entry, and reception/lobby area. Careful consideration is given to alternative entrances for dissimilar services such as medical ambulatory surgery and medical offices if they are to be located within the same building.

If the maternity care unit is within a hospital, the appearance of the hospital will influence people's opinion of the maternity service. Whether the hospital facility is an efficient, inviting building, a clutter of mismatched structures, or a gloomy relic of the industrial revolution will influence the image that people have of what happens inside.

In siting SRMC units on the hospital campus, many hospitals focus on renovating an existing multitransfer or LDR unit. Because their design is based on the surgical model, most conventional obstetric units do not lend themselves to conversion to SRMC facilities. Even if built within the last few decades, most maternity units reflect a 1940s design ethic with small, windowless rooms and long, straight, double-loaded corridors. Although the desire to make use of existing units is understandable, these facilities are most often found to be unsuitable for contemporary family-centered maternal and newborn care and are better converted to some other surgery-oriented use.

A suitable space for a new maternity unit is sometimes found in an underutilized part of the facility. Hospital planners had often overlooked this space—which we are repeatedly gratified to discover—because of its location away from other acute-care services. This isolation is often an advantage in that it allows a new entrance, focus, and character for the SRMC unit. Converting underutilized space is usually cheaper than remodeling an existing unit, and it allows new construction to proceed without interrupting the old unit.

In some cases, it is preferable to locate the new unit outside of the main hospital buildings because space within the hospital is not suitable for conversion to a functionally efficient or marketable SRMC unit, or because the cost of doing so would exceed the cost of new construction. In these instances, a location is sought where the SRMC service can be located adjacent to the hospital, either on its own or as part of a women's center or ambulatory surgery center. Where this is done, the new center can be bridged to the hospital for access to hospital-based services.

If designing a separate building to house the SRMC unit is not feasible, the next best option is usually to design a separate and easily identifiable entrance for maternity patients. This entrance is warm and inviting with adequate lighting and shelter from the elements. Families arriving in labor have priority parking located near this entrance—or valet parking assistance—so the mother and other significant family members are not separated upon arrival. Ideally, this entrance is the same entrance used by childbearing families attending prenatal and outpatient lactation services. Control of the designated entrance, especially after business hours, is a key concern. This entry must be secure and remain open for general access if prenatal classes are to be offered in the evening and must be accessible to patients in labor at all hours of the day and night.

If it is not feasible to provide a separate entrance, the path to the maternity center is carefully planned to facilitate quick, comfortable, and convenient ingress and egress. It is made easy for the family to find the correct entrance and the location of the maternity unit once inside the facility. Frequently, hospital admission for childbirth may be the family's first experience in an acute-care hospital. Some women may arrive ready to give birth, and others may have medical emergencies. Their needs, and those of family members accompanying them, require special attention. However, it is important to remember that most expectant mothers are not sick. The sight of common hospital equipment such as anesthesia machines, stretchers, intravenous pumps, and infant incubators can be upsetting to the expectant family. Walking through a busy emergency room or trauma center can be very disturbing for the family.

Reception

The interface between the maternity center and the outside world is the reception area. It func-

tions as an inviting entry/reception point to the SRMC unit and is the first line of security of the SRMC service (Figure 5-8). The reception area serves the birthing unit and the other services supporting it or located with it. Therefore, it may serve a maternity unit, a family/visitor lounge, an education center, lactation resources, diagnostic services, women's health services, ambulatory surgical services, a medical office suite, and other services.

Reception serves as an information and control area, and may also provide medical records and business office functions. The first contact with the maternity unit staff is at the reception area. It is here that families seeking admission are welcomed and helped to their destination in an LDRP room or, in some services, a triage room. Because confidential medical, personal, and financial information is transacted in the reception area, privacy needs must be carefully considered. If the reception area is contiguous with a family lounge and waiting area, it should have suitable visual and acoustic screening. Depending on the size of the facility and services provided, the reception area may require private interview spaces for preadmission, financial arrangements, and other functions. In these interview spaces and elsewhere on the unit, counters, high tables, desks, and other barriers are avoided. Instead,

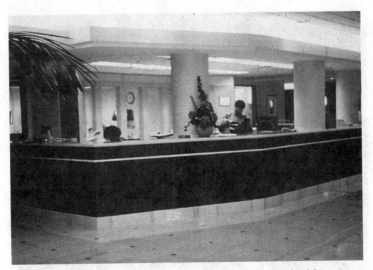

FIGURE 5–8. The reception area functions as an inviting entry to an SRMC. (Photo courtesy of Wellstar Family Birthplace, Cobb Hospital, Austell, GA.)

tables and seating arrangements are chosen for the family's comfort and to communicate a collegial relationship between family and staff members.

Family Lounge and Visitor Waiting

This area is adjacent to the reception area and close to the entrance to the birthing unit. Generally, this unit primarily serves family members and visitors of women in the birthing unit, but it may also serve people waiting to make preadmission or financial arrangements or for diagnostic or other services offered by the facility. Family visitors may need to wait at maternity units for long periods of time, often for 12 hours or more. Although one or two close family members may spend much of their time with the woman in labor, many more just want to be close at hand.

The interior design and décor of the SRMC family lounge communicate the program's service theme, consistently and uniquely providing an identity separate from other clinical services. A good model for visualizing a family lounge is an airline's frequent-flyer's clubroom. Because people may spend many hours in these places, nourishment, storage space for personal belong-ings, and seating are clustered for large and small groups and for various activities such as relaxing, snacking, reading, and watching television (Figure 5-9). The customs and needs of social and cultural groups with which the service interacts will strongly influence the design of public spaces.

Basic communication, entertainment, nourishment, and toilet needs are provided. Hot drinks and snacks are available, either free or by purchase from vending machines. Some cultures bring large extended families to the maternity facility, and may have special religious customs or dietary preferences that must be accommodated (Spector, 1995). For example, in some cultures, people prefer to bring and prepare their own food and may need access to a kitchenette to do so.

In SRMC programs, children are welcome and accommodated. This is not only to make the family more comfortable, but also to facilitate sibling involvement in the events taking place around them. A play area is provided either within or adjacent to the lounge where children's activities can be observed from the lounge or lobby. The play area has play equipment that cannot easily be taken out of the area. Public toilets, drinking fountains, and telephones placed for privacy are

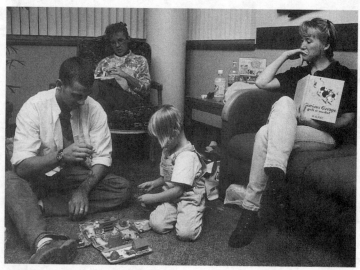

FIGURE 5–9. A family lounge and visitor waiting area. (Photo courtesy of Evergreen Hospital Medical Center, Kirkland, WA.)

accessible from the public lobby and are in close proximity to the family lounge.

Prenatal and Parenting Education Center

Having parents who understand the philosophy of family-centered maternity care, and who are emotionally and physically prepared for childbirth, is a prerequisite for a fully functional SRMC program. Without specialized education, parents will be unprepared to benefit from physiologic labor and birth management, mother–baby nursing, and other program elements that may be new to them. A comfortable and functional facility is essential for prenatal and parenting education and is also a valuable "shop-window" to the community.

Prenatal education requires facility space that is appropriate to the populations being served and available at the times that they can attend. Issues such as after-hours access, security, and nourishment are addressed in the design process, as well as the need to transform the space into a variety of teaching settings. Ideally, the education/resource center is easily and safely accessed from the main facility entrance, with access extended to evening and weekend hours. This center includes office space for educator(s) and classroom and library space with adequate storage for teaching aids and AV supplies.

In planning classroom and meeting space, both currently available and possible future programs are considered. Classroom space is designed for easy access for families and equipment, which includes a birthing bed, and the space is wired to facilitate new and future communication technologies. Storage space for personal belongings and for chairs and tables is needed in each classroom. Large, carpeted classrooms are necessary to conduct childbirth preparation classes in which the parents lie on the floor. Public toilets with infant-changing accommodations as well as a nourishment area are located near the classrooms.

Lactation Resource Center

The SRMC program emphasizes breastfeeding because it benefits the baby and also helps family development. A lactation resource center meets women's needs by providing inpatient and outpatient support for breastfeeding through information, pump rental, and retail sales. The size of the lactation resource center depends on birth volume, population served, and other factors, and can be anything from a single room for individual consultation to a multiroom center serving the needs of many women at a time.

Designs for a lactation resource center may include a reception area for clients, lactation offices for lactation consultants, a retail area for a variety of products relating to breastfeeding and newborn care, storage for pump rental, and a soiled receiving area for cleaning and processing returned pumps. A number of individual rooms or a large room divided by privacy curtains or screening is needed for lactation counseling. Each private space is adequately sized to comfortably accommodate a lactation consultant, mother and infant, support person, and necessary equipment and furniture. Lactation centers are often located adjacent to the education/resource center, thereby sharing education resources and space.

DESIGN CONSIDERATIONS FOR FAMILY CARE AREAS

Because all clinical care areas and public areas are designed to foster optimum family outcomes, the welcoming design theme of the public areas continues into the family care areas. However, the needs of the family for privacy and security are greater in the patient care areas.

Security

The presence of babies on the unit creates special control and security demands. Security needs are a major consideration that must be met without creating a feeling of exclusion or confinement in those who have legitimate access.

Although a number of useful technologies and programs are used to enhance security, the generally small number of people on each LDRP cluster and the close relationship between staff and clients are also valuable in ensuring a safe environment. Because babies remain with their mothers in the LDRP rooms and are not usually moved about the unit, this also benefits security. In facility design, careful consideration is given to controlling access and to monitoring visitors and others on the floor. Also, physician and nursing access to the unit and movement within the unit are carefully planned to ensure comfort and efficiency.

Layout of the SRMC Cluster

The heart of the SRMC system is one or more clusters of LDRP rooms. Each cluster consists of a central core surrounded by a corridor that provides access to LDRP rooms around the perimeter of the unit. Instead of moving the woman to equipped rooms, equipment and skilled personnel go to the family. The core houses the control area or communication station; areas for medication and charting; an infant holding or "respite" area; a procedure room; a nourishment station for family and staff; storage, mechanical, utility, and housekeeping rooms; and all other functions required on the unit. This arrangement centralizes nursing staff, services, supplies, and equipment for ready access to the LDRP rooms.

In addition to meeting all the requirements of clinical care, the cluster is designed for parent–staff collaboration in care and to facilitate satisfaction of the family's physical and social needs. The corridors are attractively laid out and wide enough to accommodate women ambulating in labor. Seating alcoves enable women to rest and to communicate with family members and others on the unit. Noise is reduced by the careful selection of floor coverings in corridors, proper sound insulation within doors and walls of adjacent rooms, and special wall covering in the LDRP rooms.

To provide a place for nurses and physicians to chart close to the patient's bedside, pull-down chart stations are built into each LDRP or on the corridor wall outside the room. If computerized bedside charting is selected, computer terminals and cabling are designed into each LDRP room.

Admission to an LDRP Room

Careful consideration is given to admissions occurring at different hours of the day and night.

Hospital preadmission procedures performed at an earlier date minimize the amount of paperwork at time of admission. Assessing women in LDRP rooms eliminates an extra move for those who are admitted and also avoids the need for a separately staffed triage area. A brief, initial assessment in the LDRP room before admission identifies women who are obviously not candidates for admission to the LDRP room. This eliminates the need for a triage area in most units and represents not only a more pleasant experience for families but also a substantial savings in space and cost to the organization. In a small- or medium-sized service with well-prepared parents, only occasionally will a woman not be in labor and be sent home; this is preferable to imposing a triage room and an extra patient move on every family.

Admission to a Triage Area

Although a triage area is generally best avoided altogether, in some larger services a triage area may be justified, particularly if mothers are not generally knowledgeable about the labor process and where many women come to the hospital when not in labor. The triage area is designed to be close to the communication center so its function is integrated into the staffing and operation of the closest LDRP cluster. This triage area is often the woman's first formal encounter with a hospital and is designed to provide privacy and comfort for her and accompanying family members in a nonthreatening environment.

A comfortable, reassuring environment is important for the family's sense of well-being and confidence; it can also avoid stress that could interfere with the woman's clinical condition. Maternal stress can interfere with the strength and frequency of contractions in early labor (Simkin, 1986). This could lead her caregiver to the incorrect conclusion that she is not in labor when her contractions have been only temporarily stopped by her response to her environment. Other clinical conditions such as hypertension, anxiety, and nausea are also aggravated by stress.

In triage, clinical needs are met in a nonclinical ambience. Toilet facilities; cabinets; a sink; medical gases to include oxygen, air, and vacuum; as well as the necessary supplies, furniture, and equipment are provided. Enough separate spaces are available to provide for each family's privacy and confidentiality. Some SRMC programs require a separate area for stress testing or biophysical profiles. Again, the objective is to provide privacy and create a warm, relaxed ambience; in most cases, this can best be provided in an LDRP room instead of a triage area.

THE CLUSTER CORE

Each LDRP cluster has a centrally located multifunction control/communication station. From it, all functions within the cluster are coordinated, including control into and exit from the cluster and traffic flow throughout the unit.

Control Area and Communication Station

The control area and communication station contains areas for medication preparation, physician dictation, and storage of newborn examination kits used by pediatricians to examine babies at the mother's bedside in the LDRP room. Contiguous with the nurses' station is a holding or "respite" area for newborns (Figure 5-10). Because nurse charting occurs at the patient's bedside in SRMC, nursing activity is generally less than in a conventional control area or nurses' station.

Baby-Holding or Respite Area

The facility is planned for mother–baby nursing, in which the same nurse cares for mother and baby, whether the baby is with the mother or not. In this approach to developing maternal confidence and competence, the parents collaborate with staff to ensure that both the mother's and baby's needs are met. When properly implemented, most mothers prefer to keep their babies with them in their rooms, to be cared for by both the family and their nurse.

Babies who have medical needs that cannot be adequately managed in the LDRP room are cared for in a special-care or intensive care nursery. If a well baby's mother cannot or would

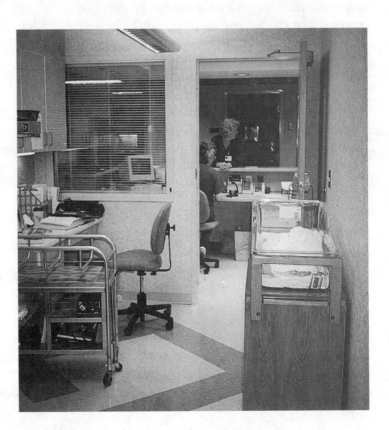

FIGURE 5–10. The baby-holding or respite area is contiguous to and accessed through the control station. (Photo courtesy of the Family Birth Place, Carroll County General Hospital, Inc., Westminster, MD.)

prefer not to have her baby in her room with her for short periods of time, the baby can be watched over in the respite area that is contiguous with the communications station. Thus, the mother–baby nurse continues to care for the baby without reliance on a nursery whether the baby is in the mother's room or in the respite area. Because entry to the respite area is through the communication station, nurses at the station control access to the respite area by visitors or guests.

Equipment and Supply Areas

The SRMC facility, the cluster cart, the powered birthing bed, and the infant stabilization bed were all specifically designed to work together for normal and emergency care in SRMC services. This equipment provides all the capabilities needed in the room, is designed to have a non-institutional appearance, and is mobile for transporting the mother or the baby out of the room if necessary. Equipment, linen, and supplies for the cluster carts and stabilization beds are located in the clean supply area of the LDRP core area. Only room supplies and routine care supplies and equipment are kept in the LDRP rooms. The cluster cart is a specialized case cart that holds all the instruments and supplies needed for managing birth. It is brought into the LDRP room when birth is imminent, and it also serves as an instrument table. After the birth, all soiled supplies and equipment are removed in the cluster cart, which is cleaned and resupplied in the core area. When properly implemented, staff should never need to leave the LDRP room for supplies, and stocking of each room is kept at the minimum necessary.

The infant stabilization bed is a special newborn warmer bed that was designed to provide all the capabilities needed to monitor and stabilize the baby, perform resuscitation or medical procedures, and also to provide a warm and secure bed for the baby at the mother's bedside. After use, equipment is returned to the dirty or soiled supply area of the unit's core for cleaning and restocking. Carts for soiled food trays, linen hampers, and trash receptacles are also returned to this area for processing.

THE LDRP ROOMS

An LDRP room provides for each woman's labor, birth, and newborn care needs. Instead of moving the mother and her baby from room to room to receive care, as in the multitransfer system, personnel and equipment come to the family, meeting their needs where they occur.

Capability

Each LDRP room is equipped to allow management and support of normal and complicated labor, birth, and recovery (Figure 5-11). Each room is equipped with a powered birthing bed that the woman, or someone she chooses, can adjust to the full range of configurations necessary to facilitate physiologic labor and birth positioning. The bed should have a cut-out opening at the front edge to accommodate upright birth. The bed should also provide positioning for instrumental deliveries or vaginal repair, including semi-Fowler, lithotomy, lateral, Sims', or Trendelenburg positioning.

Any LDRP room can be set up to enable staff to safely perform any vaginal delivery, normal or complicated, including preterm and high-risk deliveries, forceps and vacuum extractions, and repair of lacerations. All birth needs, except for surgical delivery or conditions requiring general anesthesia, are typically managed in an LDRP room. Epidural analgesia is administered. In LDRP rooms, however, general anesthesia is usually not given, primarily because of space and air change requirements. Although both of these requirements can be met by appropriate design of the LDRP rooms and their air-handling capability, cesarean deliveries and procedures requiring general anesthesia are usually performed in an operating room.

Layout

Each LDRP room has a window, a bathroom with shower or bath, a sink within the room, sufficient storage space for the family's belongings, storage space for room supplies, and a space for infant resuscitation and care. Overhead clinical lighting is unobtrusive and easily accessible and

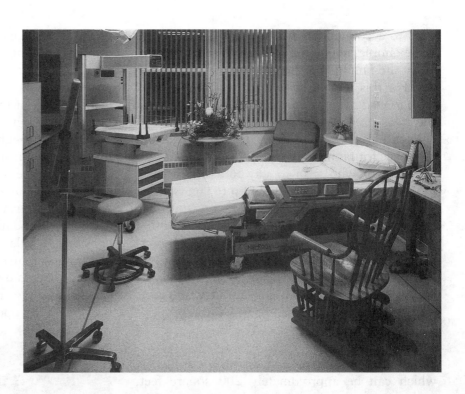

FIGURE 5–11. An LDRP room. (Photo courtesy of the Seacoast Birth Center, Anna Jaques Hospital, Newburyport, MA.)

provides surgical quality lighting for birth and for newborn examinations. Medical gases in the LDRP room include oxygen, air, and vacuum for both the mother and baby.

The LDRP bathroom should be large enough to comfortably accommodate at least two people and may include a shower, tub, or whirlpool tub to facilitate jet hydrotherapy, which has been found to increase relaxation during labor and provide pain relief. Postpartally, hydrotherapy bathes damaged tissue and increases circulation, enhancing healing and reducing pain (Aderhold and Perry, 1991). Good tub access for staff requires a large bathroom, and in some facilities tubs or whirlpool baths are located in a separate room large enough to provide access from all sides.

Use

The physical needs of the laboring mother are met by an adequate LDRP room design. This includes the need to ambulate in labor; to relax in a tub or shower; to sit, squat, and kneel; and, in some instances, to crawl. A properly designed powered birthing bed allows the woman to change position at will during labor and facili-

tates birth in the positions that work best for her. The mother may be assisted in these activities by a doula, family members, or other support persons. All of these people and activities must be accommodated in the LDRP room.

Because newborn care and most complications encountered during the neonate's stay are managed in the LDRP room, it is designed to be flexible. It has an infant care area with the capacity for any level of infant resuscitation, from simple to complex. The infant care area is located next to the mother's bed so she can observe her baby in the event of infant resuscitation needs. This clinical "zone" for the baby is closest to the door, and it provides an area for focus of clinical care activities. In SRMC care, pediatricians conduct their initial and subsequent examination of newborn infants at the mother's bedside and are provided adequate lighting, space, and equipment.

It is especially important to meet the family's social needs in the LDRP room. Childbirth and the introduction of a new person into their lives is a peak life event for the woman and her family. It is here that memories will be made that will remain with them to the end of their days. A family's social and physical needs may include the need to accommodate many people in the room. For example, many immigrant and ethnic groups value the family and the group over the individual. For this reason, large extended families may wish to visit the new mother and stay throughout the day.

Each LDRP room includes a sleeping and dining space for family members who are present for the birth or who wish to stay to assist the new mother in infant care. In addition to chairs and a table for family meals, a pull-down couch or sleeper/seat is provided for the father or other family member to stay overnight. Room appointments are similar in quality and design to those found in a hotel, with the exception of carpeting and the addition of furnishings for newborn care.

Size and Shape

Some states publish minimum areas for an LDRP, which can be approximately 200 square feet, exclusive of space for a toilet, shower, and equipment storage. It is unrealistic to expect to be able to provide adequate SRMC care in a room this small. In our experience, the room must be much larger—300 square feet or more of net space, depending on shape and other parameters—to meet the needs of clinical care and the family. A number of factors—ever-increasing consumer expectations, market competition, increase in number of personnel, the need for ambulation during labor, an increase of in-room technology, and the need to accommodate the father or other family member in the room—have led us usually to design larger LDRP rooms and suites. The actual size of the LDRP is determined during strategic planning when all relevant factors concerning room use and presentation are considered in the light of marketing and budget consideration that affect the project as a whole.

The cost of building larger rooms is not proportional to the increase in their square footage. For example, doubling the planned size of a room does not double the cost of building it. The cost of a bathroom, of fixtures, furniture and finishes, and most of the cost of construction is nearly the same whether the room is large or small. The relatively small cost saving achieved by building minimum-sized LDRP rooms is not justified in the light of having to spend years in cramped quarters that make clinical care difficult and families uncomfortable and that limit options to accommodate tomorrow's technologies and practices.

The shape of the room is also important. Particular attention is paid to ensuring the privacy of the family through room design and placement of the bed and furniture. The room has to provide sufficient space in the required directions for all the personnel and equipment needed to manage complicated birth and infant resuscitation, while also accommodating family members. Issues to consider include having room at the foot of the birthing woman's bed to allow traffic to move around the bed during the birth, and providing a clear passage for the bed to be moved through if transfer to the operating room is necessary.

DESIGN CONSIDERATIONS FOR SPECIAL CARE AREAS

The LDRP rooms are supported by a surgical suite for cesarean births and, depending on the acuity of care offered by the facility, an appropriate system for managing newborn complications. This could be as simple as stabilization capability in the LDRP room, where infants are readied for transfer to another facility, a special stabilization nursery, or a special-care or intensive-care nursery.

Cesarean Birth Suite

In general, the layout of the surgical suite is conventional except for features designed to support the family-centered mission of the SRMC program. Cesarean birth can be a particularly stressful time for the family. It is associated with fear for the well-being of the baby and for the mother, and sometimes with feelings of disappointment and failure. When general anesthesia is used, the mother will depend on the father or other family participant to share memories of the birth. These factors make it important that the surgical environment accommodates the family's social and emotional needs to the extent that it is possible.

Wherever practical, the architectural and interior design theme of the SRMC unit is carried through to the operating suite, particularly with regards to the use of color, windows, and skylights. Although access from the LDRP rooms to the surgical delivery area is designed to be quick and easy, access to the surgery suite is also carefully controlled.

Provision is made for persons accompanying the woman to change, gown, and safely store their belongings, and an infant resuscitation area is planned within each of the operating rooms in keeping with the principles of family-centered care.

Recovery Room

In small- to medium-sized maternity services, it is most efficient for postcesarean mothers to recover in their LDRP rooms. Returning the new mother to her private room provides a comfortable and familiar space to recover with her baby and family members. However, in some large-volume services, a designated cesarean birth recovery area may be required. In these instances, the recovery room, like every other area in the SRMC facility, accommodates the woman's family, including her baby, unless medically contraindicated. Therefore, in addition to all the usual recovery room capabilities, private, comfortable spaces are provided that allow newborn stabilization at the mother's bedside.

Special-Care Nursery

If it is determined that a special-care nursery is to be included in the SRMC unit, it is located close to the LDRP unit for quick transfer of stabilized sick babies and convenience for their families. As with other areas in the SRMC facility, security, architectural and interior design, as well as functional design, are directed to meeting the needs of the family and of the staff. Research documenting harmful effects on the neonate of noise, bright lights, lack of diurnal rhythm, and other environmental factors has led to many new approaches to nursery and NICU design that are carefully considered in program and design development. The baby and its family are considered as a single unit with connected needs and capabilities. In an SRMC program, family members are not visitors to the special-care nursery but are both recipients and providers of care. Provision is made for family access, comfort, support, and privacy.

Staff Area

Space for staff to change, meet, eat, sleep, and relax is located away from the LDRP clusters in a quiet area of the unit. Usually, this is "backstage" of the public and maternity care areas, in a location that is convenient to the LDRP clusters and the surgical suite. Convenient access to other parts of the unit is possible through internal circulation.

To provide the best support for families in SRMC facilities, there must be an emphasis on communication between caregivers. All maternity, pediatric, and anesthesia nurses, as well as midwife and physician providers share the same lounge. This feature is included to promote cooperation, communication, and a single-team attitude, which is helpful in caring for mothers and babies as a family unit. The staff lounge has seating clusters that provide for different activities and for privacy. The staff area includes equipped space for nursing and medical education. On-call rooms are located in a quiet part of the building near the SRMC unit, not adjacent to the staff lounge. Proximity of the on-call rooms to the clusters and the cesarean delivery suite is desirable.

For consumers, the warm, friendly, noninstitutional environment communicates that the facility cares about the families served. The design theme of the public and maternity care areas is brought into the staff areas to provide continuity of atmosphere and to communicate respect and concern for staff members as well. This is important. Often, staff members complain, "Why are the LDRP rooms so nice while we have to live with the same old sterile-looking space?" The same attention to comfort, ambience, and user needs must be applied to the spaces for staff, who spend so much time in the hospital and need a positive work environment.

EXTERNAL SUPPORT FACILITIES

Whether an SRMC unit is within a hospital or a freestanding center, it always has connections and associations with other facilities and clinical services that provide care to childbearing families. All of these services must be seamlessly integrated so that, from the family's point of view, they become part of the SRMC program and environment. Departments such as a perinatal diagnostic center, a maternal–fetal intensive care unit, or a neonatal intensive care unit are extensions of the SRMC program. Providing care that is consistent with the philosophy of family-centered maternity care, particularly as it pertains to nonseparation of the mother and father and mother and baby, requires a consistent environmental approach to meeting family needs in the external support facilities.

SUMMARY

The SRMC facility is a socially responsible design for a good family beginning in an environment that must also provide for clinical and emergency care. To fulfill the goals of the SRMC program, the needs of the family, the medical staff, and nursing staff are met without compromise to the legitimate requirements of any of these groups. Indeed, when properly executed, the design enhances the ability of these constituents to work together for the common purpose of giving families the best possible start in life.

At its introduction, the SRMC program and facility were determined by an objective evaluation process to be the best model for providing safe, satisfying, and cost-effective maternity care for the future (Kaiser Family Foundation, 1980). This determination has been validated by our experience with many SRMC programs over the past decade. Unlike LDRs and other modifications of the multi-transfer system, SRMC is not a hybrid system. It is a "pure" design that effectively supports a comprehensive care program to attain specific program outcomes.

Just as family-centered care was first implemented in maternal/newborn services and has spread into other clinical services, design that supports family-centered care is now being implemented throughout hospitals. Providing a consistent facility character and ambience communicates a hospital-wide philosophy of family-centered care to patients and staff. This character of the hospital facilities will be especially impor-

tant to young families exposed to a reassuring, participatory, and comfortable environment during maternity care. Consistency of philosophy, care, and design is important if hospitals are to capture for their other services the goodwill that is associated with an excellent experience in the SRMC program.

REFERENCES

Aderhold, K., & Perry, L. (1991). Jet hydrotherapy for labor and postpartum pain relief. *The Journal of Maternity and Child Care, 16*(2), 97–99

Basler, D. S. (1981, February). Principles of building a perinatal center. *Clinics in Perinatology, 10*(1), 9.

Beck, W. C. (1984, July). The lighting of the birthing room. *Lighting Design and Application.*

Carpman, J. R., & Grant, M. A. (1993). *Design that cares: Planning health care facilities for patients and visitors* (2nd ed.). Chicago, IL: American Hospital Publishing.

Fenwick, L. (1979). Blueprint for the humanization of American obstetric practice. In D. Stewart & L. Stewart (Eds.). *Compulsory hospitalization: Freedom of choice in childbirth.* Marble Hill, MO: NAPSAC.

Fenwick, L., & Dearing R. H. (1981). *The Cybele cluster: A single room maternity care system for high- and low-risk families.* Spokane, WA: The Cybele Society.

Flynn, J. E. (1978). Studies of the subjective influence of light and color. In Pierman, B. C. (Ed.). *Color in the health care environment.* Washington, DC: National Bureau of Standards, US Department of Commerce.

Hurst, T. W. (1966). Is noise important in a hospital? *International Journal of Nursing Studies, 3,* 125–135.

Kaiser Family Foundation. (1980). Unpublished study. Palo Alto, CA: Author.

Simkin, P. (1986). Stress, pain and catecholamines in labor. Part 1: A review. *Birth, 13,* 8.

Sisson, T. R. C. (1978). Some relationships of color and light to patient care. In Pierman, B. C. (Ed.). *Color in the health care environment.* Washington DC: National Bureau of Standards, US Department of Commerce.

Spector, R. E. (1995). Cultural concepts of women's health and health-promoting behaviors. *Journal of Obstetric, Gynecologic, and Neonatal Nursing, 24*(3).

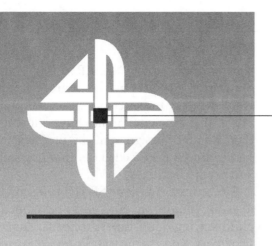

CHAPTER 6

Strategic Planning

For most established organizations, redesigning the maternity program and facility is a once-in-a-lifetime event. The birth of a new specialty women's hospital or the rebirth of an established organization's maternity service deserves consideration of all factors that could affect the facility's operation during its project lifespan.

The new SRMC service will change the culture of the organization for decades, and the new facilities should also be designed to have an equally long, productive life. Before investing millions of dollars in a new service, an organization has to consider how the in-vestment serves today's needs and also the needs of future providers, patients, and staff.

An organization's goal, when establishing a new program, is usually to improve its business and realize a reasonable return on its investment. In the case of maternity services, that goal is more complex.

First, although there are many profitable maternity services, profit is not always the primary goal. Contemporary maternity services are more often part of a long-term strategy to create and capture the greater market associated with women who direct the healthcare decision making for their families. In addition, there is extraordinary goodwill that can follow a happy family beginning, and thus gain the lifetime loyalty of young, new families to the hospital.

To meet the market development goals of the organization, a maternity program must do more than meet the standard tests of financial and market feasibility. It must also generate a level of satisfaction so high that new families will always associate the maternity facility and the hospital with high-quality, satisfying, family-centered maternity care. This happens best if the woman and her family's physical, emotional, social, and developmental needs are met by a level of care that exceeds their expectations and makes a lasting difference in their lives.

Second, maternity services are not usually freestanding. In contemporary women's healthcare, maternity is often a part of a women's service product line in a hospital, or a service of a women's center, or an element of a freestanding women's specialty "mini-hospital." Although we have focused discussion on SRMC until now in this book, when engaging in strategic planning, development, and operation of maternity care, the service must be considered within its relationship to the parent organization. In other words, the goal of a maternity service is usually tied to that of a larger organization. Therefore, creating an SRMC program requires an integrated approach to planning—linked with the master planning of the hospital or healthcare organization, and consistent with the parent organization's mission, values, and goals. In addition, where maternity is part of a women's service product line in a hospital or women's center, strategic planning for maternity will affect these services, which must also be considered.

SRMC spans a range of care from education and wellness-oriented prenatal care through emotional and social support and intervention, to highly technical acute care for women and neonates. The SRMC program is provided to an increasingly demanding and diverse clientele and spans all payer groups, and must survive and thrive in a highly competitive and evolving market. Because SRMC is a complex integration of new concepts in service, education, and marketing that can directly affect the parent organization's image and success, it warrants a more thoughtful, sophisticated level of strategic planning than is called for by other hospital services.

New facilities alone, no matter how splendid, will not ensure success. Not recognizing that the SRMC program drives and dominates facility development, many hospitals view the task in terms of bricks and mortar and focus their attention first on architectural solutions that accommodate existing attitudes and practices. In some cases, even when the organization changes to nontransfer maternity care, the facility concepts are poorly understood and hospitals build "LDRP units" that violate the basic functional, philosophical, and space requirements of SRMC.

Operational effectiveness, strategy, and strategic positioning are all essential to superior performance (Porter, 1996). Operational effectiveness means performing similar activities better than competitors. Strategy deals with the overall, long-term guidelines that are set up in an attempt to ensure the success of the institution. Positioning is how one is seen by the outside world (Ries & Trout, 1986). To be seen differently, an organization must differentiate its services from those of others, and communicate these differences in a clear and persuasive manner. Strategic positioning means performing different activities in different ways from competitors (Porter, 1998; Porter, 1996). Because strategic positioning is about carving out a niche that competitors cannot duplicate, SRMC allows progressive organizations to occupy a service high ground that is beyond the immediate reach of conventional programs.

A hospital maternity department can outperform competitors only if it can establish differences that it can sustain over time. This is not the case when hospitals simply modify existing services. For example, it is not unusual to find communities in which one hospital modifies its conventional multitransfer obstetrics unit by simply converting labor and delivery to a labor/delivery/recovery (LDR) suite or adding a few "LDRP rooms." Initially, the innovation increases market share, but it is easy to copy and easy to better. Soon, several other hospitals in the same community have improved on the first hospital's design, and the first hospital's marketing advantage is ceded to other hospitals' newer and prettier facilities.

By contrast, a unique SRMC program based on a strong philosophy and goals developed to meet childbearing consumers' needs, as well as providers' and the hospital's needs, provides sustainable competitive advantage. When a hospital converts to an SRMC program, it can serve as a magnet, attracting family-centered maternity providers and nurses from surrounding facilities. Over the years, we have seen significant instances in which family-centered SRMC programs have captured most of the more progressive providers in the area. These providers and nurses have, in turn, promoted a strong family-centered culture in their hospital. Once a facility and its staff gain the high ground in SRMC, it is extremely difficult for competitors to overtake the lead.

THE PLANNING/DEVELOPMENT PROCESS

Figure 6-1 illustrates the process recommended for planning and developing an SRMC program and facility. It is a focused process that is designed to achieve, in the most efficient and enjoyable way possible, the optimum program and facility to meet the needs of staff, families, and the organization. The process is also designed to help doctors, nurses, and administrators understand and support the SRMC program. Strategic planning can be done internally with external help as required, or a women's service development company can perform it with support from the organization.

Conceptualization

Before strategic planning begins, the parent organization is first presented with information that will allow it to become thoroughly familiar with new developments in the women's market and in maternity care. This will help the organization to

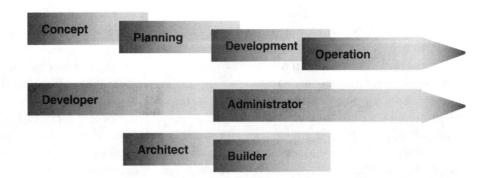

FIGURE 6-1. Process for planning and developing an SRMC program and facility.

determine interest in developing a women's health program, and maternity care in particular.

Strategic Planning

If the organization decides to proceed with strategic planning, it engages in a structured process to determine where the organization is, where it wants to go, and how best to get there. The program and facility developer, assisted by a planning team, leads the planning and development process. (For the remainder of the chapter, the term *developer* is used to signify the program and facility planning and development function whether provided by personnel within the organization or by an outside women's healthcare company.) The team represents the clinical, financial, operational, architectural, and marketing expertise necessary to guide development to meet the needs of the organization, the community, and the medical and nursing staff while preserving the integrity of the SRMC program (see Figure 6-1).

At the end of strategic planning, the organization will have a clear idea of what type of service or services it wants to provide; how big the services will be; what kind of facilities they will require; where they will be located; how they will be owned, developed, and operated; and how much they will cost to develop, build, and operate.

Development

This is where the concepts defined in strategic planning become realities. Led by the developer and a development team, all the details of the program and facility are determined and planned. During development, an SRMC administrator is selected to work with the developer in preparation

for overseeing the management of SRMC when it begins. Once defined, the building proceeds through construction drawings and construction, and staff and program development takes place so all systems are ready for the opening of the service.

Operation

An administrator is responsible for every aspect of the SRMC program, including clinical care, business operation, and marketing. In most hospitals, this executive will also have responsibility over other services, including women's services. This administrator will use the parent organization's resources as well as external resources to provide the services necessary for operating the SRMC unit. In large women's services or specialty hospitals that include SRMC, the administrator would have most services available internally. In the case of a specialty women's hospital, this administrator would be responsible for all services provided by the specialty hospital.

STRATEGIC PLANNING DESCRIBED

The strategic planning process answers three questions:

Where is the organization now?
Where does the organization want to be?
How will the organization get there?

The result of strategic planning is a plan that defines the type, scope, cost, and operation of the proposed new program and facility, and that establishes preliminary cost estimates for program and facility development and for facility construction.

A program that results in a better bottom line, improved performance outcomes, patient satisfaction, and long-term success requires strategic planning. The planning process can be a very worthwhile exercise, both for the organization and for the SRMC developers. Strategic planning helps the hospital to see itself. Then it alerts an organization to opportunities, as well as threats in the market around it. It helps focus efforts toward responding to those threats and opportunities in a constructive and structured way (Hardy, 1999).

Planning also affects operational effectiveness by communicating direction, priorities, and values to the rest of the organization. Planning guides major resource allocations, frames day-to-day decisions, motivates and energizes the organization, and enables leadership (Hardy, 1999). Planning enables the development of programs that achieve desirable goals and outcomes. To shortcut planning is to forge ahead into the unknown. A facility built without a long-range strategic plan will become no more than a memorial to today's thinking.

INITIATION OF PLANNING

A variety of circumstances may lead to the initiation of the planning process: The organization may perceive maternity care to be a way to increase or retain its share of the women's market, or as a way to attract and retain new, young families. The organization may want to communicate its commitment to family-centered care by the provision of an exemplary family-oriented maternity service. The organization may want to expand its market into new areas by building a satellite women's center with an SRMC service to capture new families who will also receive care in the parent facility. The organization may recognize that it needs eventually to relocate itself to follow its market to the suburbs, and will see an SRMC in a freestanding maternity facility as being a first step in that direction.

And then there are hospitals that have lost maternity market share to more progressive, better-positioned or better-marketed competitors, and for whom retention of a dwindling source of new families is a matter of survival.

In some situations, an organization of independent investors sees an opportunity to develop and operate a freestanding specialty women's hospital, and they may capture a portion of the women's healthcare market, with or without hospital equity participation. The development of a new breed of specialty "mini-hospitals" for women carries great potential to capture a significant share of the market for new families as well as for women throughout the lifespan. Figure 6-2 shows the Women's East Pavilion, a 28-bed, freestanding women's specialty hospital in Chattanooga, Tennessee.

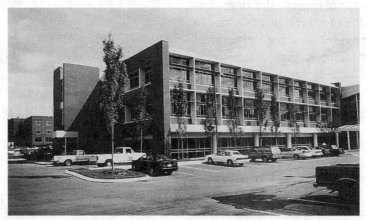

FIGURE 6–2. A freestanding women's specialty hospital. (Photo courtesy of Women's East Pavilion, Chattanooga, TN.)

PHASE I: WHERE IS THE ORGANIZATION NOW?

In today's healthcare market, it is often to an organization's advantage to align maternity services with women's health (Keile & Delaney, 1986; Lutz, 1996; Rynne, 1985), ambulatory surgery, and other services. Therefore, before strategic planning can begin, decision makers should understand the current and future maternity and women's market, national trends in maternity and women's healthcare, business and scope of women's and maternity care, and the potential for integrating women's services with maternity care at its core. Information on trends in maternity care and women's care is presented to enable leadership to understand the potential effects of a contemporary maternity program on the future of the organization, to visualize various options, and to decide whether to proceed with strategic planning.

Review of Parent Organization Strategic Plan

Unless the proposed SRMC facility is to be a completely independent, freestanding women's specialty hospital, its strategic planning will build on the plans already in place for the parent institution of which it will be part, or with which it will be affiliated. This parent organization could be a general acute-care hospital, a hospital system, or other healthcare system.

Interest in a contemporary maternity service often marks a shift in the hospital's culture or priorities. The hospital's strategic plans are reviewed to ensure that the development of new services is consistent with national trends and new developments, with the business objectives and strategies, and the organization's culture and philosophy. In this review, the current positioning of the organization is assessed along with the current women's and maternity programs and facilities. During the strategic plan review, it is common for information to be presented that alters perceptions of where the institution should be headed relative to women's services and maternity care.

Current Program Assessment

This assessment gives a clear understanding of the organization's existing situation. It consists of a comprehensive study of market dynamics, payer environmental and financial data, as well as clinical program and facility for maternity care. Conditions that influence present and future provision of maternity care are assessed. The facility's strengths and weaknesses, opportunities and threats (SWOT) are analyzed. Information is developed about present and future markets, and also about providers and payers. In addition to examining the facility's current clinical programs, management structure, facilities, and business operation, it is important to determine the organization's culture and philosophy of care.

The assessment includes a review of provider and program sensitivity to childbearing women and their families, comparison to "best practices," and determination of what stages the organization is currently experiencing in the transition to contemporary family-centered practices. Current clinical and nursing attitudes and skills are assessed, as well as provider and staff willingness to learn about and provide the SRMC program of care.

Market Dynamics

The strategic assessment is to gain a thorough understanding of the maternity marketplace and how the current or to-be-developed clinical maternity program and providers fit into that picture. The process begins with an assessment of "market dynamics," which consists of market area demand projection, market area demographic trends, market share analysis, payer influences, provider influences, and competitor effects.

Competitor Analysis

Completing an assessment of competitors' maternity programs helps to identify potential threats to the hospital's position and to its stated goals. Consumer research and review of competitive marketing materials also furnish information about the specific features of each hospital's maternity program. Through this process, it is possible to develop at least an intuitive sense for the competitors' current strategies and their strengths and weaknesses (Porter, 1998).

Consumer Preferences

This phase of planning may include qualitative and quantitative consumer research. No organization should undertake a large capital investment without first ascertaining consumer preference by one or both techniques (Braus, 1997). The "voice of the consumer" must be captured and heeded as part of the planning process.

Focus groups are an excellent means of obtaining qualitative information. Focus groups explore consumer receptivity to the strategies under consideration and provide an open forum to explore current service product issues in more depth. They are also an excellent way to capture current perceptions of provider attitudes and practices.

Over the past 7 years, we have conducted numerous focus groups concerning "women's wants" in every geographic region of the United States. Using moderator scripts and group-depth interview technique, the key factors have been identified, including facility and program components that women value. Reports of focus groups totaling 500 women (Phillips & Fenwick, 1999a) indicate that women consistently rated compassionate, friendly nurses as the most important element of maternity care. As one woman put it, "I don't care how much money they put into a facility. If you don't have caring nurses, you can forget it." Another finding was a strong preference for programs that did not disrupt early family care by transferring the family to a postpartum unit. Research further supports that the quality of nursing support has profound effects on the woman's satisfaction or lack thereof with her childbirth experience (Fowles, 1998; Simkin, 1991; Wilcock, Kobayashi & Murray, 1997).

Although focus groups can lead to a greater understanding of consumer preferences, they are necessarily limited to relatively few participants. Ascertaining the overall voice of community women with any degree of confidence requires large-scale consumer survey research. Telephone surveys are useful to gather the opinions of a large number of women about their preferences for maternity care. However, some care is needed in the survey research design. Telephone and other surveys that measure existing consumer preferences without their knowing what is possible in the future may be of little value in determining what women will respond to when new programs and environments are available for them to see.

For example, in the 1980s, some hospitals asked women if they would prefer to remain in the room in which they gave birth or go to the postpartum unit. Most visualized the technical, cold, and uncomfortable delivery room that was their only experience in those days, and chose to leave it as soon as possible. This was interpreted as meaning that there would be little demand for LDR rooms. However, once comfortable birth and recovery environments were made available, the same population group previously "surveyed" showed an immediate and strong preference for this environment.

Today, we have a similar situation when women are asked if they would prefer an LDR room or an LDRP room. Having no knowledge about an SRMC facility's environment, but having a general idea of a labor and delivery unit's noise and bustle, some may choose LDR and postpartum rooms over LDRP rooms in the belief that changing rooms would result in a quieter, more comfortable environment for postpartum care. Overall, well-designed consumer research can provide essential information to planners interested in and capable of funding the random survey. However, it must be kept in mind that a random survey of current attitudes and preferences represents no more than a starting point from which to develop community awareness of, and interest in, SRMC.

Market Area Analysis

Analysis of the market area is part of the environmental (external) analysis that comprises the strategic planning process. The market analysis seeks to answer four essential questions regarding maternity services:

Where do the consumers (families) who deliver at my hospital originate?
How many potential consumers are there?

How many births are there today, and how many will there be in 5 years?

How many consumers are delivering at my hospital rather than at one of my competitors?

The Maternity Service Area

The maternity service area is the geographic area from which consumers originate. This area may be considerably different for maternity than for the hospital overall. Because most women will have only one or two children in their lifetime, they want the experience to be the way they have always dreamt it will be. Therefore, they do not hesitate to drive significant distances to get the kind of program/service/physician that they want. This expectation, coupled with the fact that the majority of expectant women are healthy, means that the maternity service area may be more extensive than the hospital's traditional service area.

Childbearing Women

As part of the market area analysis, it is important to know how many childbearing women live in the service area and how many are projected to live there in 5 years. They are the members of the population who will be supporting the SRMC program!

Projected Number of Deliveries

The projected number of deliveries is obtained by applying the area fertility rate to the number of childbearing women in the area. (In this book, we are using *fertility rate* to mean the number of births per 1,000 women aged 15 to 44. This measure is different from a *birth rate*, which is the number of births per 1,000 persons in the total population.) The resulting product is the projected number of deliveries or "size of the market." This is essentially the size of the "pie" that all area hospitals will fight over for market share.

Number of Consumers at Competitor Hospitals

At this writing, 17 states collect and report to hospitals origin/destination data. The "origin" part of the data is the number of deliveries in each zip code or county (origin). The "destination"

part is the hospital at which the delivery occurred. The resulting distribution permits the computation of market share for each hospital. In those states where data are not collected by the state, share computation is more complicated and a variety of informal methods must be used. Once data are collected, resulting share is used as a basis for status quo projections and for building growth models to project future deliveries.

Payer Environmental Analysis

Today, health insurance plans influence women consumers' selection of a physician and choice of facility for maternity care. Women often select a plan when they are planning to become pregnant or during early pregnancy so they can have the hospital or care provider they prefer. Therefore, hospitals in managed care markets must make themselves as appealing as possible to their consumers (Braus, 1997).

To best position itself, a hospital should understand how payers see the hospital and the impact of managed care plans on the hospital's market. The hospital also should analyze the financial impact of each payer on obstetric performance. A comprehensive analysis of payers and their actual as well as potential financial impact on the hospital is required.

Financial Analysis

Historically, maternity services have sometimes been viewed as "loss leaders." Spending heavily on resources to improve or design a new maternity program without at least a break-even scenario may not be justified, even when other contributions to the parent organization are considered.

A thorough financial analysis includes a review of reimbursements by payer, contribution margins by diagnosis-related group (DRG) and by provider. The staffing costs by nursing unit are also analyzed. The key point to remember during the strategic planning phase is that the financial contribution of any hospital program may be a key component in decision making about new facilities, renovation, or program restructuring. No internal analysis can be complete without a financial review performed by a fiscal expert with a clear understanding of the revenues and costs associated with the maternity program.

Clinical Program Review

The existing maternity care program and facility are assessed to determine where it is relative to defined stages of maternity care development. These stages of the Maternity Transition Scale are shown in Box 6-1.

Current practice is an important indication of the amount of change that will be necessary to develop an SRMC program. However, the amount of change needed is not as critical to successful program implementation as are the attitudes of the maternity care providers, nurses, and hospital management. If these groups are enthusiastic about implementing a family-centered maternity care program, the change process is likely to be smooth. Deep and widespread resistance forebodes a difficult and expensive change process and may be reason to abandon plans to change from the existing multitransfer system. In these instances, it may not be feasible to upgrade the maternity facility at all, and development should be confined to interior design and program enhancements.

Maternity Transition Scale

The tables in Box 6-1 are used in making initial assessments of the existing status of maternity programs and facilities and for quantifying the degree of change necessary to achieve the benefits of an SRMC program:

- Facility design is in transition from the multitransfer model to SRMC.
- Medical practice is in transition from routine procedures to evidence-based, normalcy-oriented labor, birth, and newborn care.
- The nurse's role is expanding to provide for all stages of maternal/newborn care and to provide education to support family beginnings.
- Newborn care is transitioning from nursery-based care to mother-baby nursing.
- Support for family-centered care is growing and is spreading beyond the maternity service.

- Maternity service organizational and management structure is consolidating.
- Family education is in transition from a limited number of classes to comprehensive programs that support family development.

Identifying the stage that the organization is currently in is extremely useful in planning for change to SRMC. Priorities can be easily noted and appropriate plans made to help the current program transition to SRMC.

Program Data Analysis

Program data analysis is conducted as part of the strategic assessment phase to compare the program against benchmarks for all medical diagnostic category (MDC) 14 (maternity) cases. The result is to establish outcome targets, such as average length of stay and cesarean rates, that become proxies for quality and reduced cost of operations. One way that costs are affected is through facility sizing, which depends on decisions about outcome targets. Developing outcome targets for SRMC requires an understanding of practice changes that influence outcomes. For example, as previously discussed, many of the components of normalcy-oriented childbirth management are associated with reductions in clinical procedures such as cesarean birth.

Program Staffing Analysis

Personnel staffing cost is the most significant component of a maternity service's direct cost. Therefore, to project future staff costs, it is necessary to review the current maternity program's staffing and budget and to develop the maternity staffing budget under a future project program with assumptions for volume, case mix, and average daily census.

From a nursing management perspective, staffing analysis includes three distinct components:

- Analyzing staff requirements, in full-time equivalents (FTEs) and dollars
- Analyzing staff schedules (daily, weekly, and so on) that include individual shift assignments by planning period

BOX 6 – 1

Maternity Transition Scales

A. Facility Design

Stage 1   A multitransfer unit with separate rooms for admission, labor, delivery, recovery, postpartum, and newborn care.

Stage 2   A multitransfer unit with birthing rooms or LDR rooms in addition to labor and delivery rooms. There is a nursery for well-baby care.

Stage 3   A multitransfer unit with a suite of LDR rooms replacing the labor and delivery rooms. There is a nursery for well-baby care.

Stage 4   A multitransfer unit with LDR rooms and a mother–baby postpartum unit for mothers and their babies. There is no well-baby nursery.

Stage 5   A SRMC facility with clusters of LDRP rooms to provide labor, birth, and postpartum/newborn care in one room.

B. Medical Practice

Stage 1   Little support for or participation in childbirth education process. Care during labor and birth characterized by routine medical interventions and minimal flexibility. High rates of operative intervention. Babies are sent to a nursery from the delivery room.

Stage 2   Provision of some education regarding the events of childbirth and hospital routines. Flexibility regarding routines such as IV fluids, confinement to bed, EFM, regional anesthesia, lithotomy position for delivery, episiotomy, and so forth. Some physician participation in education programs.

Stage 3   Participation in providing education to prepare women for the events of childbirth and postpartum. Flexible in the application of unit routines. Ambulation and position changes allowed during labor when they do not interfere with planned medical interventions. Education directed toward imparting information about hospital policies. Limited interest

on the part of medical staff in reducing rates of medical intervention.

Stage 4   Support for the provision of education for women to allow them to take an active role in the events of childbirth. Some support for physiologic labor and birth management and mother–baby nursing. Value of family support during labor acknowledged. Some initiatives in place to reduce induction, episiotomy, regional anesthesia, and cesarean section rates. Mother–baby care is available.

Stage 5   Integration of education in all aspects of prenatal and inpatient clinical care. Universal support for normalcy-oriented labor, birth, and newborn care. Staff encourages family involvement in all aspects of maternal and newborn care. Emphasis on integration of childbirth education into clinical care throughout pregnancy and inpatient stay. Low induction, episiotomy, regional anesthesia, and cesarean section rates. Active support for mother–baby care.

(Continued)

B O X   6 – 1   *Continued*

Maternity Transition Scales

C. Nursing Care

Stage 1   Nurses educate women about hospital routines and unit policies and provide care in keeping with routine physician orders. Separate staffs for normal newborn nursery, labor/delivery, and postpartum units. Staff shared among units in extreme situations.

Stage 2   Nurses educate women about the events of childbirth. Somewhat flexible in application of patient care routines. Separate staffs for normal newborn nursery, labor/delivery, and postpartum areas. Some staff cross-training to allow "floating" or occasional rotation of staff between units.

Stage 3   Nurses provide education for all women in preparation for the events of childbirth and postpartum. Ambulation and position change encouraged throughout labor and birth. The importance of mother–baby care emphasized. Separate staff for labor/delivery. Integrated staff for mother–baby unit. Some rotation of staff between these two areas.

Stage 4   Nurses educate women to empower them to take an active role in the events of childbirth and involve family in all aspects of clinical care. Staff are prepared educationally and experientially to work in either labor/delivery or mother–baby unit, but typically work in only one area.

Stage 5   Nurses integrate education in all aspects of clinical care and support normalcy-oriented care during labor, birth, and the newborn period. Integrated staff of nurses competent to care for well newborns and maternal patients in all stages of antepartum, intrapartum, and postpartum care.

D. Newborn Care

Stage 1   Infants admitted to and routinely cared for in newborn nursery. Visitation to mother according to set feeding schedule or on specific request. Minimal regard for the developmental needs of the infant or family.

Stage 2   Infant receives care in newborn nursery but can spend prolonged periods of time with mother on her request. Some attention paid to infant's developmental needs in planning care. Care provided by newborn nursery nurse regardless of location of infant.

Stage 3   Infants admitted to mother's room. Emphasis placed on acknowledging infant's developmental needs while in mother's room. Routine infant care provided in mother–baby room by a single nurse. Infant returns to nursery for examination by pediatrician and care at night.

Stage 4   Infants admitted to nursery or mother's room. Routine infant care provided in mother–baby room except at night or when mother asks to have care provided in nursery. Emphasis on providing infant care in keeping with developmental needs of infant.

Stage 5   Care of infant fully integrated with care of mother, in a single location. Regard for the developmental needs of the newborn forms the basis for all newborn care. All aspects of infant care provided in a setting that promotes family involvement.

(Continued)

BOX 6–1 *Continued*

Maternity Transition Scales

E. Family-Centered Maternity Care

Stage 1 Standard clinically oriented unit management.

Stage 2 Some accommodation to FCMC at unit level.

Stage 3 Strong commitment to FCMC with appropriate practices.

Stage 4 Strong commitment to FCMC principles and practices with administrative support.

Stage 5 Hospital-wide family-centered care with exemplary FCMC program.

F. Organizational Structure

Stage 1 Maternal–newborn services are under the direction of separate obstetric and pediatric departments. OB is further divided into separate labor/delivery and postpartum. The management structure of the pediatric department is further divided into NICU and normal nursery units.

Stage 2 Labor/delivery and postpartum areas are managed as a single unit. NICU and nursery are each separate units.

Stage 3 Labor/delivery, postpartum, and newborn care areas are managed as a single unit. NICU is a separate unit.

Stage 4 Labor/delivery, postpartum, newborn care, and NICU are managed as a single service.

Stage 5 A single newborn–maternal service with authority over ancillary services provided to maternity and newborn patients.

G. Education Programs

Stage 1 Limited number of classes designed to impart knowledge of hospital routines and physician preferences.

Stage 2 Classes designed to instruct women about reproductive anatomy and physiology, the events of childbirth, and hospital routines for maternal and infant care.

Stage 3 Limited curriculum of childbirth education programs prepares women for childbirth and the postpartum period. Program emphasis is on pain management. There is emphasis on breastfeeding.

Stage 4 Curriculum of childbirth education programs prepares women to take an active role in their care during childbirth and the postpartum period. Emphasis on physiologic labor and birth, nonpharmacologic pain management, and mother–infant care.

Stage 5 Comprehensive program of childbirth education sponsored jointly by hospital and medical staff prepares women and their families to assume an empowered role in planning conception, pregnancy, childbirth, and the first years of parenting.

- Analyzing staff allocation to meet acuities and patient care needs on a "real time" basis with fluctuating obstetric demand

Using a sample budget projected for an idealized SRMC program, this information is used to discern opportunities for improvement when doing the financial modeling. Budgets for labor and delivery, postpartum, and newborn nursery are combined into one in SRMC.

Facility Review

A thorough facility review initiates facility design for a new SRMC program. The facility review begins with a review of the hospital site master plan, a review of all current space use, and a review of the hospital's current maternity care facility. Particular attention is paid to all areas on the hospital campus that could possibly be used for a new maternity care program. The facility review includes equipment and capacity analysis as part of strategic planning for facility design.

In light of the current surfeit of hospital space nationwide, existing space is carefully considered before seeking new construction solutions. These space resources are sometimes realized as shelled space, or they can be found as hospitals close inpatient bed units. Often, this relocation benefits the clinical services that are moved and also frees up space suitable for a contemporary maternity service.

Contemporary maternity designs do not usually fit into spaces occupied by conventional maternity services. For a number of reasons, including the surgical orientation of multitransfer obstetric units, their frequent location in less-desired windowless parts of the hospital, and the physical configuration of the obstetric space, it is usually less expensive and better in the long run to make a fresh start somewhere else. A new location also allows the old unit to function during transition.

Strategic Assessment Report

The outcome of phase I of strategic planning is a report that addresses the existing strategy and describes the current program's environment and situation. The report presents results about care programs, provider practices, facilities, operations, and consumer education. This report presents viable options for both program and facility changes and makes recommendations for action plans. In the case of a proposed new freestanding specialty women's hospital, the report provides information necessary to decide whether to proceed, and what type and size of services to offer. At this point, the organization selects whether to continue interest in a new maternity service. If the answer is yes, financial models are developed for one or more program and facility options.

PHASE II: WHERE DOES THE ORGANIZATION WANT TO BE?

In entering phase II, the organization has made a decision to proceed with planning for maternity or maternity and women's services, and has an understanding of the program and facility options available. Unlike planning for a new suite of operating rooms, for example, where the basic operational principles are understood and agreed on, planning a contemporary SRMC program requires that the planners first understand new concepts and then select from these concepts to develop a program and facility that will best meet the organization's long-term needs. The developer presents these SRMC and women's healthcare concepts to the organization and its planning team.

Creating a Shared Vision

Development of a contemporary maternity program requires the participation and support of all the groups on which its success will depend. Peter Senge writes that the preeminent leadership function in successful organizations is to inspire its members with a shared vision of the future they seek to create. He explains that directives from on high will never succeed (Senge, 1990). This is certainly true in planning SRMC. All staff members and care providers must understand and buy into the care model. In the case of a proposed new specialty hospital, where there is only a group of investors and as yet no staff, the task of creating a shared vision is far more straightforward. However, because of the greater influence that each participant can have on the venture's success, it is particularly important to ascertain that a shared vision has been achieved.

Program/Facility Planning Team

A planning team is assembled that brings together all the necessary business, medical, nursing, design, marketing, and management skills. This requires that the developer collaborate with the organization (or owners in the case of a freestanding facility). The team is multidisciplinary, knowledgeable, influential, and supportive of the philosophy of family-centered maternity care and facility design and the hospital's strategy. The developer leads the planning team, which typically includes representatives from the organization's executive and financial management team, clinical programs, facility planning, marketing, community advisory board, and the architect.

Physician Leadership

Successful maternity programs depend on informed and progressive medical staff working collaboratively with the development team to ensure development, implementation, and maintenance of the highest quality program. To accomplish this goal, physicians must actively participate in every aspect of decision making when planning the new clinical service (Moore & Komras, 1993). Physician support or lack thereof can make or break a program.

Physician Involvement in Planning

To gain cooperation from physicians when planning and developing the new maternity program, the way physicians think, what motivates them, and the pressures under which they work must be considered. Understanding these factors enables the organization to design and implement a maternity care program that meets physician as well as family needs. Physicians today feel beset on all sides. The movement from a fee-for-service model to managed care and capitated payments has created a bureaucratic headache for physi-cians that threatens their incomes (Kongstvedt, 1995). To maintain their income, many physicians have had to increase the size and pace of their practice, working harder and longer hours (Marcus, 1995).

Physicians today worry increasingly about attracting and retaining patients (Moore & Komras, 1993). Managed care may make it difficult to maintain a steady patient load as patients switch from plan to plan. Managed care plans and hospitals may also be seen as increasing competition for patients by recruiting additional physicians or favoring the use of midwives, family practitioners, or nurse practitioners. In addition, managed care and our litigious society have reduced physician autonomy. At one time the sole determinants of medical care, physicians are more and more constrained in their medical decisions by outside agencies in the name of cutting costs or reducing liability exposure.

Other factors have also eroded the traditional role and status of the physician. The media have been vocal about the high cost of healthcare and the financial rewards of physicians. The consumer movement has made patients more likely to question their doctor's judgment and seek second opinions. Patients feel less loyal and are more likely to "doctor shop." The ever-present specter of malpractice suits also increases physician stress and damages the doctor–patient relationship.

Considering all of this, from the physician's point of view, being asked to assist in designing and implementing a new maternity care program can be seen as all drawbacks and no benefits. It may be perceived as yet another criticism of medical practices to a group already experiencing a siege mentality. If the new program plans to incorporate additional or alternative care pro-viders, it can be viewed as introducing unwelcome competition for patients. The inevitable meetings will take valuable time from an already overcrowded schedule. Finally, change requires that individuals who are used to being the authorities, acting independently, and getting quick results work as team players on a project that may take years to come to fruition (Rice & Keck, 1984).

It is largely because of many of these stresses that some physicians have established new freestanding healthcare facilities. A physician-owned specialty hospital is seen as providing a degree of financial and professional practice independence not available in conventional maternity services. In some cases, physicians have been frustrated in their attempts to provide better services for their patients in hospitals that are unwilling to change, and they see practice and financial benefits in carving out women's healthcare and maternity care from unresponsive multispecialty hospitals. In other cases, hospitals have joined with physician investors to establish jointly owned facilities that avoid duplication of services.

Determining Motivators

To gain their cooperation, hospital-based physicians must be helped to understand the benefits of the hospital's plans on the medical practices and the quality of patient care. Rice and Keck, in *Persuading Physicians* (Rubright, 1984), cite two generic motivations why a hospital's planning should be of interest to physicians.

Commitment to Improved Patient Care

The first motivation is "commitment to improved patient care." Physicians want to provide quality care for their patients, which includes getting the best possible care for their hospitalized patients. This requires a top-notch hospital staff, up-to-date facilities and equipment, and a first-rate program. Involvement in program planning for a new obstetrics service gives physicians the opportunity to influence equipment purchases, facility renovation or construction, and improvement in nursing staff and support personnel. This should result in higher quality, more cost-effective, more patient-responsive care (Rice & Keck, 1984).

Enlightened Self-Interest

The second motivator is "enlightened self-interest." Because hospitalized patients perceive their care as a single experience, the impression the hospital makes will affect perception of the physician's care. Physicians benefit by association with high-image hospitals. If a hospital is seen as an attractive place for patients, market share for both the hospital and the physicians who practice there will increase.

Involvement in program planning can benefit physicians in planning for their own practices. They can gain useful information about community needs, marketing strategies, and so forth. They can help shape hospital recruitment policies so they minimize adverse impact on patient share or even create new income opportunities.

Maximizing Physician Participation

Because program development and implementation can be lengthy, interest can fade. Physicians are encouraged to stay with the process by frequent, clear, and concise communications from the developer and hospital staff. Meetings are conducted with sensitivity to the time constraints of physicians. Scheduled at a time convenient to the physician, they are planned to start and end on time and last an hour or less. There is a formal agenda, and leaders use an issue-oriented technique when conducting meetings. Because physicians are action oriented, all meetings include progress reports. Measurable successes help physicians to stay with the process (Rice & Keck, 1984).

Project planners also keep medical staff in other departments informed about the project. If other department staff perceive that the maternity service is getting undue attention and budget to their detriment, the success of the program can be threatened. This can be forestalled if other department staffs understand that women usually determine where their families get health care (Braus, 1997). If women are pleased with the hospital's maternity care services, they will develop loyalty to that hospital. Thus, a healthy maternity service contributes to the overall well-being of the hospital and, eventually, to all of the medical practices.

Working in collaboration with the developer, a physician champion can be pivotal in bringing about the type of future-focused thinking needed for change to occur. This physician leader must be committed to the vision and understand the changes that need to be made in the organizational culture. Because of the extensive amount of time required for the change process, the hospital often compensates the physician leader's position.

Consumer Advisory Board

Including consumer input in designing new maternity programs helps staff understand parents' needs and desires for the childbearing year. Input gathered by conducting focus group research during the strategic planning process can be valuable in assessing attitudes and preferences of members of the community representative of the maternity program's target market. A consumer advisory board provides a forum for ongoing discussion with members of the community regarding the hospital's maternity services.

An advisory board can broaden the hospital's perspective regarding community attitudes and needs for maternity care as well as strengthen relationships with the community of childbearing families. The consumer advisory board can also help the hospital staff to be better listeners. Through dialogue, both consumers and providers can gain a better mutual understanding. Finally, a consumer advisory board can help the hospital develop and maintain a program, services, and policies that are family-centered and consumer-based (DePompei, Whitford & Beam, 1994).

Architect Participation in Program/Facility Development

The organization and the developer should jointly select the project architect. A new SRMC unit represents an important opportunity for the hospital to define its progressive, family-oriented mission to the community, and this justifies a special effort to seek out an architectural firm that can translate the hospital's vision into an inspiring, functional, comfortable, and welcoming facility. It is important to stipulate that the developer (who functions as the hospital's or owner's representative) directs the architect to ensure that the architect does not bias the process toward conventional maternity care programs. This is particularly important when the architect's experience is primarily in designing multitransfer LDR systems. If the architect has not previously designed a functional SRMC unit, he or she should participate in all planning team activities related to learning about SRMC. During the planning process, state licensure, JCAHO, and other regulatory/accreditation requirements must be carefully considered. The architect participates in the development of the facility functional and space plan, assists with site selection and overall layout of spaces, and provides advice concerning state and local regulations and compliance with laws, regulations, and special code requirements. In some instances, current regulations may not reflect an understanding of mother–baby nursing, and variances or updating of the regulations may be necessary.

Becoming Informed

After the planning team has been assembled, it must become knowledgeable about all aspects of women's programs and contemporary maternity programs and facilities as they affect the organization. During this process, information is gained about service, facility, business, and marketing options available to the organization. During this phase of strategic planning, the organization develops a common understanding and vision for its future women's and maternity services. This is achieved through presentations by the developer and also by providers and clinicians experienced in contemporary maternity care, by review of the literature, by site visits, and through participation in a vision retreat.

Service Options

Depending on the results of the assessment, the organization might pursue one or more of the following service options:

1. *Provide multitransfer maternity care in a multitransfer setting using an LDR suite and a separate postpartum unit.* A conventional multitransfer service can be remodeled by the consolidation of labor, delivery, and recovery rooms into LDR rooms. Because this does not require remodeling of the postpartum or nursery areas, this is often the least expensive alternative to build. As described below, using LDR rooms does not require the introduction of a new nursing staffing model, and is usually the easiest for staff to accept.
2. *Convert an existing maternity service to SRMC.* A conventional multitransfer system

or a multitransfer LDR system can be converted to an SRMC service. This generally requires remodeling of the labor, delivery, and recovery area, of the postpartum unit, and of the nursery, staff, and public spaces. Where the location, window exposure, access, and space shape or "footprint" of the facility is suitable for SRMC, this may be a good option. However, building a new SRMC facility often yields a better result and may be more cost-effective than remodeling a space more suitable for a surgery-related use. In converting to SRMC, medical and nursing staff development is a more significant issue than it is in a multitransfer LDR service.

3. *Provide a new maternity service in, or adjacent to, the hospital.* This could be a new multitransfer system that uses LDR rooms or a new SRMC facility. The advantages and disadvantages of these LDR rooms and SRMC are discussed later in the chapter. There may be strong advantages for building an SRMC service as part of a new women's center. The new service could be built into, onto, or next to the hospital buildings, with bridge, tunnel, or other connections to hospital services. This approach would allow sharing of common services and spaces, and facilitate the creation of a family-centered environment distinctive from the rest of the hospital.

4. *Provide an off-campus maternity service either as a hospital-owned, joint-ventured, or independent venture.* A satellite multitransfer LDR or SRMC facility design could be part of an off-campus women's center. Ambulatory surgery, diagnostic, and other services could be part of this off-campus women's center. Alternatively, the maternity service may be an element of a freestanding women's specialty "mini-hospital." A medical office building may be part of either a women's center or a women's specialty mini-hospital.

Maternity System Options: LDR Rooms or SRMC?

In deciding whether to design an LDR suite or commit to an SRMC program and facility design, the organization has many factors to consider. The planning team must understand these factors, as outlined below.

LDR Rooms

Building labor/delivery/recovery rooms consolidates the functions of separate labor, delivery, and recovery rooms into one room (LDR) while retaining separate rooms for postpartum and newborn care. Building LDR rooms is a simple architectural solution that will increase patient satisfaction (Figure 6-3). It does not require

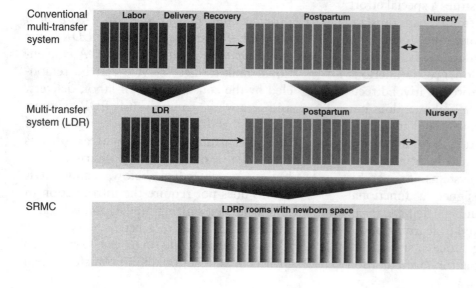

FIGURE 6–3. LDR suite. LDR suites consolidate the separate labor, delivery, and postpartum portions of the multitransfer system.

philosophical, attitudinal, or cultural changes on the part of management, medical, or nursing staff. Neither does the use of LDR rooms require significant changes in nursing or medical staff practices. LDR rooms preserve the basic multitransfer system divisions of maternity care into labor/delivery, postpartum, and nursery areas. Modifying a multitransfer system by building LDR rooms does not require nurses in existing services to learn new skills.

When building LDR rooms, the hospital can still use the existing postpartum private and semiprivate rooms and the newborn nursery. In some communities, hospitals have even retained old postpartum units that require families to share rooms and bathrooms with other families. Because the use of LDR rooms does not require nursing staff to have skills necessary for the full range of clinical care, comprehensive staff development and education in family-centered maternity care is an option, not a necessity for operation. Requiring only that the medical and nursing staffs learn how to deliver babies in an LDR room instead of in a delivery room, the basic conversion to care in LDR rooms can usually be accomplished at the departmental level and at minimal cost.

We do not mean to imply that LDR rooms preclude a family-centered approach to care. There are excellent family-centered maternity care programs provided in some hospitals with separate LDR suites, nursery, and postpartum units, which use three different nursing staffs to provide care. Some hospitals with LDR rooms have combined mother and baby care by converting postpartum and well-baby nurseries into mother–baby nursing units. In these instances, there are two nurse managers and two nursing staffs: labor, delivery and recovery, and mother–baby.

SRMC

The SRMC program drives facility design and operation. SRMC is a comprehensive program that provides family-centered care based on a nontransfer model of care that brings support, services, and equipment to families who remain in the same room throughout a normal maternity stay. The SRMC program has specific goals

beyond a safe environment for the mother and baby, which include the promotion of confidence, competence, and family development. The SRMC maternity program, not the facility design, is the bigger factor in determining the successful operation of the service.

Skill Requirements

The SRMC program requires that all nurses have knowledge and skills in family-centered maternity care, including labor and birth management, postpartum and newborn care. In addition, the goals of the SRMC program require nursing and provider attitudes and practices intended to give the family the best possible beginning. Although family-centered goals, attitudes, and practices are important wherever maternity care is provided, they are more critical to the success of SRMC programs than they are to multitransfer LDR programs.

Staffing Requirements

The multitransfer LDR system typically requires three nursing staffs to provide birthing, postpartum, and newborn care. This requires more FTEs than a single, multiskilled staff because maternity care is characterized by wide fluctuations in demand, particularly in the labor and birth segment of care. LDR suite census, for example, can vary from zero to overload within the span of a single nursing shift. Unless the staff is multiskilled, each of the three units must be staffed at a level high enough to handle peak loads that may occur during any shift. When the additional staffing required to handle peak loads in each of the three areas is added up, the multitransfer service requires more nursing FTEs than in an SRMC program in which multiskilled nurses can shift care to wherever peak loads occur.

Moving the mother from an LDR suite to a postpartum unit and the baby from the LDR room to a nursery adds a further nursing care requirement. Each transfer requires a discharge nursing assessment of mother and baby, which has to be documented and communicated to the postpartum and nursery staff; transferring the woman and her belongings and the baby; and an admission nursing assessment by the postpartum and the nursery staff, which must also be documented. A study revealed that this process usually takes between 1 and 1½ hours per transfer of mother and baby (Phillips & Fenwick, 1999b). Each time a new room is used, it also requires that the room be cleaned and resupplied. Each transfer requires discharge assessment and documentation, reporting, admission assessment and documentation, and cleaning time. When these requirements are totaled for mother and the baby and multiplied by the number of transfers that take place each year, just LDR to postpartum and nursery transfers alone can account for additional FTEs in maternity services.

Space Requirements

Because SRMC uses multipurpose LDRP rooms for the entire stay, fewer rooms are needed than with systems that use special-purpose LDR and postpartum rooms. Although the advantages of the SRMC facility over a multitransfer LDR facility become less pronounced as the number of births increase, SRMC is always more efficient in

function and space use even in very large maternity services (see Chapter 5).

Quality of Nursing Care

High-quality, family-centered maternity care can be provided in either SRMC or multitransfer programs. However, it is easier to provide in SRMC because there is continuity of nursing care that enables the maternity nurse to respond to family and newborn care needs personally identified during the labor and birth process. Rapport, trust, and empathy established by the nurse during labor and birth continue into postpartum and newborn care. Subtle impressions about the family's clinical or psychological status are not lost during transfer of care to another nurse, and a source of communication errors that could arise in the transfer of orders and treatment plans is also avoided. The transfer process does not disturb the family during the highly significant first hours of meeting and getting to know their baby (Figure 6-4). Infection control is facilitated by SRMC because it reduces the number of contacts between the family and different rooms, different

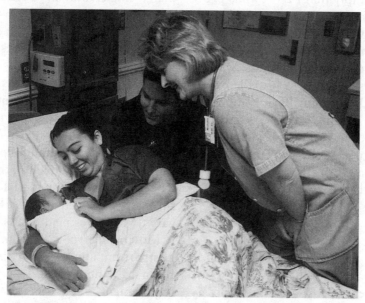

FIGURE 6–4. A family. Rapport, trust, and empathy developed by the nurse during labor and birth continue on to postpartum and newborn care. (Photograph courtesy of Evergreen Hospital Medical Center, Kirkland, WA.)

beds, and different staff members. Lastly, patient and staff injury, a common occurrence during transfer, is avoided.

Startup and Operating Costs

The SRMC program may cost more to develop and operate during the start-up period than developing and operating a multitransfer service with LDR rooms. This is because of SRMC's need for a design of comprehensive program and extensive staff development. However, once implemented, SRMC staffing is more efficient than staffing for systems that require transfer. When it is staffed correctly, SRMC requires fewer FTEs than the same level of care provided in a multitransfer LDR system. The staffing level required is, in the long term, the most important factor determining the cost of a service. Unlike development and construction costs, which are one-time expenses, the cost of extra staff members required by an inefficient program and facility design continues year after year and will ultimately far exceed the cost of developing an effective program and facility.

Because of its more flexible room use, the SRMC facility often requires less space than a multitransfer LDR facility. This should be assessed for each situation, because facility geometry can determine this. In general, however, a new SRMC facility tends to be comparable to or less costly than a new multitransfer LDR facility.

Decision Making

Although there are many advantages to SRMC, there are also many reasons that an organization may want to develop a multitransfer unit with LDR rooms. Although some reasons are valid, other often-stated reasons have no basis in fact and stem from a reluctance to take on the organizational and developmental challenges of implementing a new program.

Reason #1

The organization or key stakeholders do not support the philosophy or goals of SRMC. The organization is not willing to invest the time and money to convert its medical and nursing practices to family-centered care, particularly when this includes unfamiliar concepts such as mother–baby nursing, physiologic birthing, and family participation in care. Building LDR rooms may be the only feasible option in this situation.

Reason #2

The only available space cannot be converted to an SRMC facility. Occasionally, the existing maternity unit is in a building that cannot feasibly be converted to an SRMC facility, and there is no other space available anywhere else on the hospital campus. In these situations, building LDR rooms into an existing labor and delivery unit may be the only option available that will improve the environment for families and staff.

Reason #3

The hospital may only be able to afford to remodel or redecorate the labor and delivery area. However, in considering total costs, program and staffing inefficiencies of operating a multitransfer unit must be considered, because these may, in time, negate any savings from a more limited construction project.

Reason #4

The hospital may believe that "The birth volume is too large for SRMC," or that "We cannot convert to SRMC because we have a tertiary-care service serving high-risk families." These are not valid reasons. Although the physical space needed by large birth volumes may have to spread into multiple spaces, sometimes not even on the same floor, this is more of a liability in a multitransfer LDR unit than in an SRMC acuity gradient (as described in Chapter 5). In the multitransfer LDR unit, every mother has to be moved off the LDR unit after birth, sometimes to a distant postpartum area. In the SRMC acuity gradient, however, only women who have cesarean births have to be moved—all others remain in an LDRP room. When lack of space requires the unit to spread to another floor or to a distant location, this location can serve as a step-down unit for postsurgical or antenatal care.

Best Practice Site Visits

Planning for the future can benefit from knowledge of what is possible in the present. An effective way to break through mental barriers to change is to make site visits to hospitals where successful maternity programs can be seen in action. Programmed site visits to successful maternity services help physicians and hospital staff understand program and facility concepts that are part of the models being considered. These site visits are not quick trips to see a facility design or physical layout. An experienced facilitator accompanies site visitors, explains the program in detail, and identifies the program and facility strengths and weaknesses (Crompton, Maisenbacher, Eppley & Phillips, 1999).

To prepare for the site visit, the developer gives each participant articles from the literature on family-centered maternity care, implementing change, LDR services, mother–baby nursing, SRMC, and team building. Each participant also receives documentation (a workbook) that outlines the key features of the program to be visited and provides a structured format for site visit observations and interviews, including core questions to help structure the participants' assessment of each site.

At the conclusion of the visit, the facilitator leads a discussion and summarizes the day's activities and observations (Crompton et al., 1999). Participants refer to the observations recorded in their workbooks when making decisions about the maternity program under consideration at their home organization. Extrapolating from the best of what was observed, site visitors begin to envision what might be possible in their own situation (Barrett & Cooperrider, 1990).

The Vision Retreat

Vision retreats are an integral part of the planning process. The retreat does not take place until after the planning team has become knowledgeable about all aspects of women's care, SRMC, and the program and facility options available to

the organization. The goals of the retreat are to reach consensus and to affirm:

- The philosophical nature of the maternity service
- Mission, vision, and positioning statements
- Consensus on the program and facility model for the maternity service

Vision retreats usually take place at a comfortable site or neutral ground away from the hospital. As explained, this retreat is scheduled only after considerable education and dialogue have occurred and site visits have been completed.

Philosophy

A philosophy for an institution, department, or program is a "belief" statement that directs people in the organization in the achievement of their purpose. Beliefs and values as well as depth of understanding about an event determine to a great extent how people think about a situation. During the vision retreat, representatives of all affected groups—physicians, midwives, nurses, ancillary staff—agree upon a philosophy of family-centered maternity care. All policies, procedures, protocols, standards of care, job descriptions and staff selection and evaluation methods are based on this philosophy. A philosophy also provides the basis for decision making about care provided for families during the childbearing year. The new philosophy is integrated at every level of operational policy. All staff members, including and especially top management, are expected to carry out their work in a manner consistent with the mission and vision statements. (See Box 6-2 for a summary of the steps in developing a new maternity program.)

Mission

The mission statement for the maternity service is built on the mission of the parent organization. It articulates the deeper reasons for the maternity service's being and the promise it holds for improving the lives of families. The real test of a successful mission lies not in its words but in whether the people who work for the organization know, feel, and fulfill its spirit (Dow &

BOX 6 – 2

Process for New Maternity Program Development

Parent organization's mission and goals
⇩
Program's purpose, scope, and type
⇩
Maternity service's mission and goals
⇩
Shared vision of how the program can be developed and implemented
⇩
Focused program and facility development
⇩
New maternity program
⇩
Quality outcomes
⇩
Achievement of program and organization's goals

Cook, 1996). In other words, the mission statement describes the core ideology or values of the program and explains why it exists.

The mission should not be confused with business strategies, which may change with the times. Strategies are the methods an organization uses to accomplish its purpose or mission. Strategies that have succeeded in the past may not continue to succeed in the future. Strategies must be continually rethought. Core ideology, however, will remain the same. It may never be fully realized, but it serves as the ultimate, constant goal.

Shared Vision

In addition to stating the hospital's core ideology, the women's or maternity program must develop a shared vision for the future (Collins & Porras, 1996). This vision addresses what the maternity department wants to become (Page, Sagely & Midgett, 1995). This shared vision serves as the driving force for changing an existing maternity program or developing a new one. It is also essential for designing the facility to house the program.

Many leaders have personal visions that are never translated into shared visions capable of inspiring organizational change. Vision statements developed by a leader or leadership team without input from the rest of the organization's members are seldom translated into action. A genuine commitment to change requires that the key stakeholders communicate their vision, incorporate input from others, and build a common "picture" of the future (Senge, 1990). This process is the next step of a vision retreat after the development of a mission statement.

Vision statements reflect the unique situation of each program and facility. Box 6-3 provides examples of vision statements that were developed by hospital planning teams using a consensus process.

Positioning

A vision retreat also focuses on development of a positioning statement. This statement answers the question, "How do we want to be seen by our customers?" (Ries & Trout, 1986). Positioning or branding crafts a maternity service's image so consumers can differentiate and choose among

BOX 6 – 3

Examples of Vision Statements

- Our SRMC program will be a comprehensive program of physical, psychosocial, and developmental support during the childbearing year that results in families that are bonded, nurturing, and enduring.
- Our hospital will become a center of excellence for childbearing women and their families. Our birth center will provide a full spectrum of care and will be a model for others.
- Our hospital will be recognized as the preeminent regional perinatal referral center, a site of academic excellence, offering a comprehensive range and depth of maternity care services to women of the area. Our hospital family-centered maternity service will be the standard by which other area providers are measured.

hospitals. For example, one hospital may position itself as a high-tech perinatal center; another might want to be identified as the good neighbor, family-friendly birth center. Ideally, an organization selects a positioning statement that reflects mission and competencies, is not currently occupied by a competitor, and cannot be easily duplicated by competitors.

The positioning statement also should reflect attributes valued in the marketplace and serve as the basis for all promotional activities for the clinical service (Gombeski, 1998). To be effective, it must be founded on actual clinical practice and the real strengths of the service. If the hospital does not deliver on the promise it makes to the community, promotional and marketing campaigns will ultimately fail. The positioning statement is intended for internal use only and is not meant to be disseminated to the public.

Philosophy, mission, vision, and positioning statements provide the foundation for all clinical care, facility marketing, and resource allocation decisions that follow. This firm foundation becomes the central focus around which questions are asked and answered as the maternity program develops.

The Product Design Framework

The outcome of the second phase of strategic planning is the planning team's answer to the question "Where does the organization want to go?" These parameters are described in a detailed product design framework (PDF). From its research, the organization has the information to choose options in the best interest of the organization, of the community, and of medical and nursing staffs. It can determine whether it wants to provide a multitransfer LDR or an SRMC service; if it wants a new maternity facility or prefers to remodel the old; or if it wants to provide maternity alone or in conjunction with women's health or other services. The organization may select to build an SRMC service as part of a women's center or as a component in a specialty mini-hospital for women.

PHASE III: HOW WILL THE ORGANIZATION GET THERE?

Once the product design framework has been established, there may be questions that remain to be answered. How will the new maternity service relate to the other hospital services? Will the service make financial sense? Will the organization be able to receive the necessary approvals for the project? Will the community support the project? How much will it cost to develop the programs? How much will it cost to design, engineer, and build the facility? If there is more than one facility option, which is the most functionally and financially feasible?

During phase III, planning moves from concept development to concept definition and feasibility. At the end of phase III of strategic planning, the developer provides the organization with all the information needed to proceed with development.

Sizing the Maternity Facility

Space planning for the clinical areas of a maternity service begins with determination of the number of LDR and postpartum rooms needed in a multitransfer facility, or the number of LDRP rooms needed in an SRMC facility.

Information gained during the earlier market, program, and facility assessment is used in sizing the maternity facility. The most significant parameters are (1) present and potential market, (2) admission and discharge patterns, (3) length of stay, and (4) referral patterns.

Normative Comparison

Birth projections are determined by the assessment of the maternity service area and the market area analysis described earlier. However, birth volume must be translated into total obstetric discharges, which include undelivered discharges, to be useful in determining room requirements. Normative DRG data for patients discharged from MDC 14 (pregnancy, childbirth and puerperium) are available from the National Center for Health Statistics (NCHS). These data list patient discharges by DRG (370 through 384) and the days of care provided to patients discharged from each DRG. However, both the occurrence rate of practice-dependent DRGs such as cesarean sections and the average length of stay (ALOS) of maternity patients must be adjusted according to projected differences in the current and future clinical practices.

Admission and Discharge Patterns

Comparison of admission and discharge patterns, with normative hospital data of similar size and patient population, may reveal information about current practice. If, for example, the incidence of discharges from a particular DRG was significantly higher than national or regional norms, inappropriate practice patterns may be present. If, on the other hand, discharge rates are much lower than other hospital norms, unmet need may be present. Because the ALOS of cesarean delivery patients is typically 3 or more days, the cesarean delivery rate anticipated in the new program significantly influences the need to build and operate postpartum obstetric beds or LDRP rooms and other inpatient facility resources.

The rate at which patients are admitted to the obstetric unit and are subsequently discharged without giving birth is also of special interest. Typically, the number of patients discharged without giving birth ranges from 5% to 15% of the birth-related discharges. This rate, however, is highly dependent on community education and clinical practices, and these factors must be considered in attempting to predict future rates.

Average Length of Stay (ALOS) Comparison

ALOS significantly influences inpatient facility requirements. The NCHS publishes a yearly summary of ALOS data on a national and regional basis. The report, part of the National Hospital Discharge Survey (NHDS), is based on a random sample of hospital data. However, the LOS of SRMC care may differ significantly from national averages, particularly if a normalcy-based labor

and birth management program is successfully implemented.

Referral Patterns

Analysis of referral patterns is of relatively little importance in maternity care except when planning for a tertiary-care service operating in multihospital environments. Referral pattern analysis involves patient origin studies to determine the place of residence and travel distances of patients discharged from a hospital. Referral pattern analysis is particularly applicable for regionalized care concepts.

Planning Methodology

Three planning techniques are frequently used to determine obstetric room and bed requirements, normative models, simulation models, and mathematical models.

Normative Models

Normative models have the advantages of being easy to apply and needing little data input. However, these models have the disadvantage of being based on historic practice in a system different from the systems being considered. For this reason, their helpfulness is limited.

Simulation Models

Simulation models, in contrast, provide a wealth of occupancy information, but these models require substantial investment of time and resources. Simulation models require a sophisticated, real-world understanding of what actually happens on a maternity unit, and also understanding of how community education, clinical practices, and unit policies in a future program will change what happens.

Mathematical Models

One input into the development of an accurate simulation model is information derived from mathematical models of room requirement. The mathematical model that we use is the Poisson process, which has been shown to be a particularly straightforward and efficient approach to establishing baseline parameters useful for obstetric facility planning.

Accurate simulation requires the parameters to be adjusted depending on community, market, practice, and other characteristics. Accurate simulations of room requirements are as much an art as a science.

The Poisson Process

The Poisson process was developed from probability and queuing theory. Use of this model requires data input on the arrival rate (the expected number of admissions or births per time period) and service rate (ALOS). Given these data, the Poisson process predicts unit occupancy. However, this process is applicable to obstetric facility planning only if several important conditions are met:

- The admissions must represent rare events with only a small portion of the population hospitalized at any time.
- The admission of one woman is independent of the admission of any other woman.
- Admissions must be random events independent of season, day of week, and time of day.

The Poisson process assists in weighing elements of construction costs, average facility utilization (occupancy), and the risks of being filled to capacity and its related requirement to house "overflow patients" in alternative locations.

Any interference with the randomness of admissions could potentially alter the accuracy of the calculation of the number of rooms required. All maternity admissions are not random. For example, there is diurnal variation in the onset of labor and also predictable peaks and valleys related to time of year. Events that can interfere with random admissions include any scheduled admission for cesarean delivery, antepartum hospitalization, induction of labor, or other similarly nonrandom procedure. If a significant proportion of admissions is scheduled and not random, use of the Poisson process will inaccurately estimate

the number of LDRPs actually required. Even in the best-managed situations, a certain amount of provider-induced clumping of admissions related to time of day and day of week has to be accepted. These factors need to be quantified and applied to the results of the Poisson process in order to create an accurate simulation.

Wherever the continuum of care is provided in a separate location, such as an antepartum unit, LDR suite, or postpartum unit, the Poisson process needs to be applied to the determination of room requirements in each of these units. It will be found that each division of the facility substantially increases the total number of rooms needed.

The Turnaway Probability

This is used to determine what number of rooms represents a suitable trade-off between maximally utilized space such that all LDRPs are full and some patients (turnaways) must be cared for in some less desirable alternative space, and the alternative of having underutilized rooms. The appropriate number of LDRP rooms must strike a balance between the desire to meet demand and avoid patient turnaways with the requirement to utilize these expensive inpatient resources.

SRMC Clusters

In the case of an SRMC facility, dividing the number of LDRP rooms by the number of rooms in each SRMC cluster yields the number of clusters needed. The appropriate number of rooms in each cluster depends on the acuity of care to be provided and other factors (see section entitled Acuity Gradient in Chapter 5). The acuity and character of care, as well as the number of LDRP rooms, will determine the type and size of facilities needed in the cluster core and also the overall size of each cluster.

Staff area size is generally proportional to the gross size of the clusters, but other factors such as subspecialty care or the need to serve ambulatory surgery or other services must be considered. Space requirements for public areas such as an education and resource center, family lounge, and other facilities are also affected by numerous factors including location, birth volume, community preferences, and marketing goals.

Special-Care Nursery

In determining the need for a special-care nursery, the strategic planning process considers long-term needs for neonatal services in relation to the organization's goals and the availability of resources in the area. Analysis of data regarding neonatal services considers historic utilization patterns, normative comparisons, design and utilization options, the effect of mother–baby nursing on the maternity unit, and future market demand for neonatal services.

Planning for Success

It is possible that an SRMC program's ability to attract from surrounding markets may exceed the most optimistic projections by a wide margin. Particularly when the SRMC is in a large metropolitan area, nearby communities may respond to the SRMC program by coming to the program from outside of the hospital's original maternity service market area. This can more than double the volume of an SRMC service over the original market projections. Unless the need for expansion had been considered during planning, the service may not be able to add enough capacity to the facility to meet the higher birth volume while maintaining a nontransfer care program for all families.

Ownership Options

As new specialty hospitals for women ("mini-hospitals") are being developed and operated, joint ownership arrangements are being created. These usually include hospitals, physicians, and nonphysician investors. Freestanding specialty hospitals for women are also being developed and operated by investors and without any hospital ownership participation.

Development and Operations Options

Organizations have several options to create the SRMC model. These include developing the

maternity program and facility internally, using outside resources as needed, or contracting with a women's healthcare development and management company to develop and manage the program and facility for them. This decision depends on the skills, resources, and time available in the organization to learn about and develop an SRMC program.

Most hospitals that have renovated multitransfer units by the addition of LDR rooms have done this internally, using either a local hospital architect or architectural firm with expertise in LDR room design. The hospital staff is usually able to convert medical and nursing staff practices to use of LDR rooms.

In contrast, implementing SRMC is a significant challenge, usually requiring outside expertise. A comprehensive staff development program requires an investment of financial and staff resources that may not be available. Hospitals may prefer to contract with a women's healthcare company to develop staff skills and attitudes and to serve as an external resource for later operation.

SRMC services can be hospital operated and managed, hospital operated but managed by a specialty maternity care provider, operated by a joint-venture partner, or operated by a women's healthcare company with expertise in SRMC. Having a single point of overall responsibility for planning, development, and operation provides consistency throughout the process.

Financial Modeling

Before approving a concept design for SRMC, the organization must test the financial feasibility of proceeding with the project as defined. Capital costs and clinical operating assumptions must be integrated into a unified model to assess the impact of the proposed change. Financial modeling is an absolute requirement for this important analysis.

At the conclusion of the strategic planning phase, the organization's executives will understand in broad terms what must be done, how it could best be done, and what various options would cost. Options selected by the organization are developed at this stage to include cost estimates and preliminary financial models of projected business performance. This information is then fed into an interactive financial model to test various "what-if" scenarios and determine the most financially viable alternatives.

FACILITY AND PROGRAM DEVELOPMENT BUDGET

The costs associated with the development of the new program and/or facilities are generally capitalized along with architectural, construction, and equipment costs. This means that the overall project cost budget should include an estimate of the development costs. Examples of budgets for a new SRMC service and for a freestanding women's specialty hospital are illustrated in Chapter 7, Figure 7-1.

PROGRAM AND FACILITY DEVELOPMENT SCHEDULE

A Gantt chart is used to plan the program and facility development schedule. The Gantt chart illustrates the integration of the multiple planning, development, and implementation functions necessary to bring the facility "on line."

SUMMARY

The strategic planning process is the essential first step in moving toward a contemporary family-centered maternity care program. During phase I of the planning process, the organization answers the questions: Where are we now? Where do we want to go? How do we get there? The process involves identification of current strengths and weaknesses and plans for taking maximum advantage of opportunities.

At the conclusion of phase II of the strategic planning process, the organization should have a clear idea of the type of program and facility it envisions for the future. A product design framework (PDF) is prepared.

By the end of phase III, a business and operational model has been selected and defined for development. The organization has a clear idea of what type of service or services it wants to provide; how big these services will be; what kind of facilities they will require; where they will be located; how they will be owned, developed, and operated; and how much they will cost to develop, build, and operate.

REFERENCES

Barrett, F. J., & Cooperrider, D. L. (1990). Generative metaphor intervention: A new approach for working with systems divided by conflict and caught in defensive perception. *Journal of Applied Behavioral Science, 26*(2), 219–239.

Braus, P. (1997). *Marketing health care to women.* Ithaca, NY: American Demographics Books.

Collins, J. C., and Porras, J. I. (1996, September-October). Building your company's vision. *Harvard Business Review, 74*(5), 65–77.

Crompton, D. A., Maisenbacher, R., Eppley, G. Y., & Phillips, C. R. (1999). Changing workplace, changing minds. *Nursing Management, 30*(2), 47–50.

DePompei, P. M., Whitford, K. M., & Beam, P. H. (1994). One institution's effort to implement family-centered care. *Pediatric Nursing, 20*(2), 119–121.

Dow, R., & Cook, S. (1996). *Turned on: Eight vital insights to energize your people, customers, and profits.* New York: Harper Collins.

Fowles, E. R. (1998). Labor concerns of women two months after delivery. *Birth, 25*(4), 235–240.

Gombeski, W. R. (1998, Fall). Better marketing through a principles-based model. *Marketing Health Services,* 43–48.

Hardy, G. (1999). Why *not* plan? *The Navigator* [online newsletter]. Available at **www.hsmg.com/article2.htm**.

Keile, R. L., & Delaney, P. E. (1986, May). Should you consider a women's center? *Health Care Strategic Management.*

Kongstvedt, P. R. (1995). *Essentials of managed health care.* Gaithersburg, MD: Aspen.

Lutz, S. (1996, March 11). Universal opens first in chain of women's hospitals. *Modern Healthcare, 26,* 22.

Marcus, L. J. (1995). *Renegotiating health care: Resolving conflict to build collaboration.* San Francisco: Jossey-Bass.

Moore, N., & Komras, H. (1993). *Patient-focused healing: Integrating caring and curing in health care.* San Francisco: Jossey-Bass.

Page, C. W., Sagely, L. S., & Midgett, D. M. (1995). *Transformation and strategic management: Shifting the paradigm.* Oxnard, CA: Graham Page.

Phillips, C. R., & Fenwick, L. (1999a). *Focus group summary.* Scotts Valley, CA: Author.

Phillips, C. R., & Fenwick, L. (1999b). *Transfer cost study.* Scotts Valley, CA: Author.

Porter, M. E. (1998). *Competitive strategy: Techniques for analyzing industries and competitors.* New York: The Free Press.

Porter, M. E. (1996, November-December). What is strategy? *Harvard Business Review, 74*(6), 61–78.

Rice, J. A., & Keck, Jr., R. K. (1984). *Motivating and sustaining involvement in persuading physicians: A guide for hospital executives.* Rockville, MD: Aspen.

Ries, A., & Trout, J. (1986). *Positioning: The battle for your mind.* New York: McGraw-Hill.

Rubright, R. (1984). *Persuading physicians: A guide for hospital executives.* Rockville, MD: Aspen.

Rynne, S. (1985, Fall/Winter). The women's center: A bold strategy. *Hospital Management Quarterly,* 12–17.

Senge, P. M. (1990). *The fifth discipline: The art and practice of the learning organization.* New York: Currency Doubleday.

Simkin, P. (1991). Just another day in a woman's life? Women's long-term perceptions of their first birth experience. Part I. *Birth, 18*(4), 203–210.

Wilcock, A., Kobayashi, L., & Murray, I. (1997). Twenty-five years of obstetric patient satisfaction in North America: A review of the literature. *Journal of Perinatal Neonatal Nursing, 10*(4), 36–47.

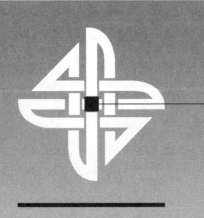

CHAPTER 7

Single-Room Maternity Care Development

As described in Chapter 6, strategic planning answers the questions "Where is the organization now?", "Where does the organization want to be?", and "How will the organization get there?". Continuing this approach, development can be described as "Getting the organization to where it wants to be."

The goal of program and facility development is to create a functional program and facility that meets the requirements of the organization's strategic plan. This plan defines what services are to be developed, how they are to be provided, what size they are to be, how they are to be marketed, what type and size of facility is to be built, where it is to be built, and who should lead the development. It also establishes a budget for development and implementation of the program, and for facility design, engineering, and construction. Examples of a preliminary budget and a Gantt chart are illustrated in Figures 7-1 and 7-2. A Gantt chart is a planning tool that details how the development components are to be integrated and implemented.

As discussed in Chapter 6, the strategic plan may call for the new maternity service to be part of a larger program that may include women's healthcare, diagnostics, surgery, and other services. When this is the case, program and facility development for all related services is led by the developer and team to provide seamless integration of programs and facility. However, for clar-

ity, only the maternity component will be discussed in this chapter.

THE DEVELOPMENT TEAM

A program and facility development team lead the process. For continuity between planning and development, it is desirable that the development team contains several members of the planning team responsible for the development of the strategic plan. However, the function of the development team is different from that of the planning team. Instead of exploring and defining new options, the development team must develop the program and facility defined in the clinical program and facility plans. The development team should represent clinical, financial, operational, architectural, and marketing expertise necessary to guide the process required to meet the needs of the organization, the community, and the medical and nursing staff, while preserving the integrity of the SRMC program.

THE DEVELOPMENT PROCESS

It is critical that the development team understands the goals and operation of an SRMC

Surgery/SRMC Center Budget

24	LDRP Rooms	18,000	Square Feet
6	Bed Special Care Nursery	3,000	"
4	Operating Rooms	7,200	"
10	Inpatient Med/Surg Beds	4,800	"
	Diagnostic Center/Imaging	4,800	"
	Education/Resource Center	9,600	"
	Bldg Support, Lobby, Admin	18,000	"
15.00%	Grossing Factor	9,810	"
	Total Square Footage	**75,210**	"

Construction Cost Per Square Foot		$	200

	%	
Land Acquisition & Site Development	**4.59%**	1,000,000
Building Construction	**69.08%**	15,042,000
Architectural Design Fees	**4.84%**	1,052,940
Equipment	**9.18%**	2,000,000
Program and Staff Development	**4.50%**	979,957
Developer/Owner's Representative	**0.90%**	195,991
Contingency	**6.91%**	1,504,200
Total Project Cost	**100.00%**	**21,775,088**

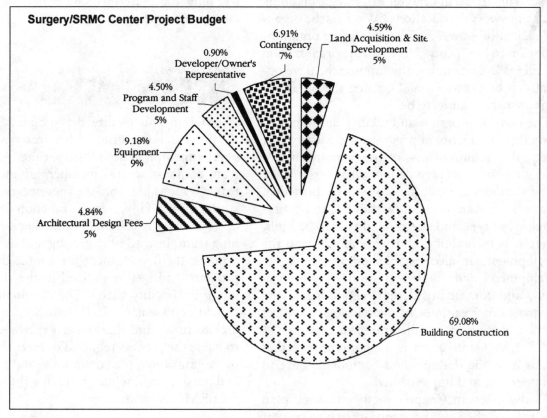

A

FIGURE 7–1. (*A*) An example of a preliminary project budget for a women's specialty mini-hospital with ambulatory surgery. (*B*) An example of a preliminary project budget for an SRMC renovation.

SRMC Renovation Budget

24	LDRP Rooms	18,000	Square Feet
6	Bed Special Care Nursery	3,000	"
2	Operating Rooms	3,600	"
	Education/Resource Center	9,600	"
	Bldg Support, Lobby, Admin	12,000	"
15.00%	Grossing Factor	6,930	"
	Total Square Footage	53,130	"

Renovation Cost Per Square Foot $ 110

	%	
Building Renovation	62.39%	5,844,000
Architectural Design Fees	4.37%	409,000
Equipment	21.35%	2,000,000
Program Development	4.72%	442,000
Owner's Representative	0.94%	88,000
Contingency	6.23%	584,000
Total Project Cost	100.00%	9,367,000

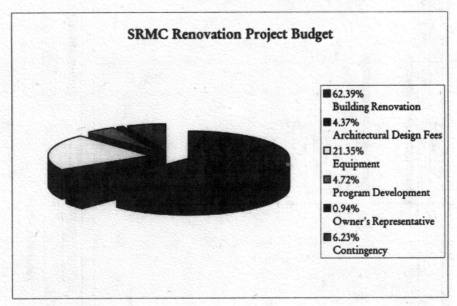

SRMC Renovation Project Budget

- 62.39% Building Renovation
- 4.37% Architectural Design Fees
- 21.35% Equipment
- 4.72% Program Development
- 0.94% Owner's Representative
- 6.23% Contingency

B

FIGURE 7–1. *Continued*

program, and also supports the organization's mission and goals for the maternity program. Sometimes, key positions on a development team are given to powerful opponents in an attempt to get "buy-in" from them. Giving development authority to anyone who is not willing to support or fully understand the program and goals of SRMC is unwise and can result in the program and facility being compromised.

Development takes place in two stages. In stage I, all the details of the program and facility are determined and planned. During this stage, the administrator is appointed to work with the developer in preparation for managing the SRMC program when it begins. In stage II, construction drawings are prepared and the facility is built. During stage II, the SRMC program development continues to be ready for implementation when the facility opens.

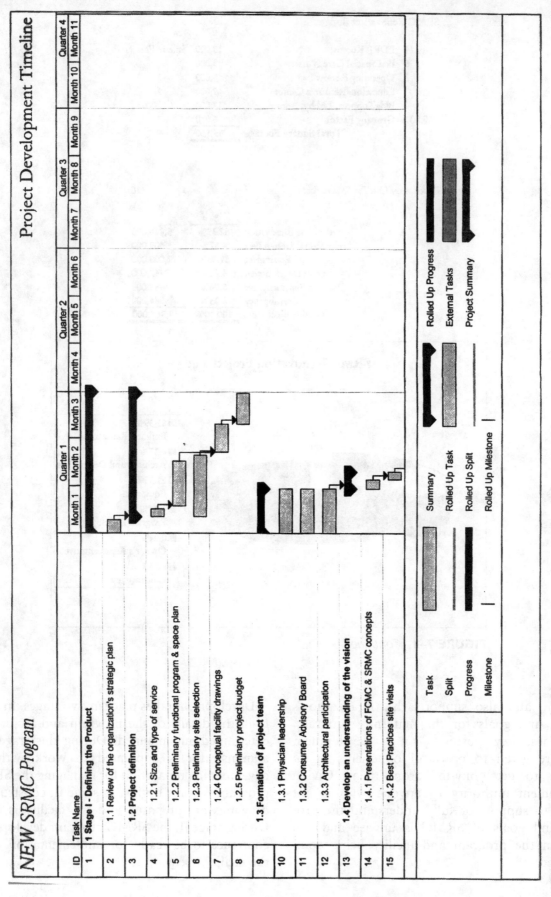

FIGURE 7-2. An example of a Gannt chart.

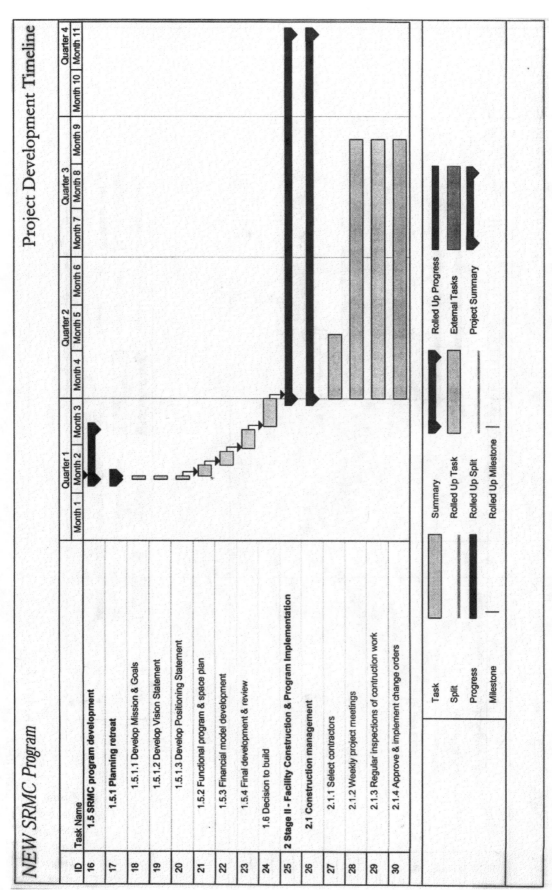

FIGURE 7-2. *Continued*

FIGURE 7–2. *Continued*

THE PROGRAM DEVELOPER

Whether an organization is converting a conventional obstetrics unit into an SRMC program and facility or starting up a new SRMC service, the program and facility development process requires a skilled, dedicated, strong "product champion" who will direct and take responsibility for the entire project. Planning for a successful SRMC program and facility requires a broad range of expertise in the women's healthcare business, plus proven strengths in the planning, development, design, construction, and operation of SRMC programs. In addition, the developer position requires critical judgment and insight into the direction of future developments in maternity and women's healthcare. Ideally, the program developer also has a strong background in business, financial management, marketing, and program/facility development.

Whether the position is filled by a person in the organization or contracted through a healthcare development and management company, the developer reports to the organization's chief executive and has responsibility over all aspects of the development, including clinical, marketing, and architectural input. The developer provides guidance, structure, and process. It will be up to the developer to define and communicate the organization's vision for maternity care, make trade-offs, and forge fit among activities. The developer's essential skills include the ability to resolve conflicts, build consensus, and empower others to achieve results (Trofino, 1995). This leader must be able to clearly articulate SRMC and the organization's vision for the future, inspiring others with that vision.

During program development, the mission, goals, strategies, and action plans identified in the strategic planning process are implemented. The developer functions as an "owner's representative," ensuring that every aspect of program and facility design and construction supports the program goals.

THE ADMINISTRATOR

If a women's healthcare company is to manage the SRMC service on behalf of the owners or par-

ent organization, an administrator is appointed to prepare for taking over administration when the development process is completed. Depending on the program's scope, the administrator may or may not have additional responsibilities to other services.

If the SRMC service is to be administered by the parent organization, the organization's administrator and the developer work as a team during development. Ideally, SRMC (and associated services, if there are any) should be organized as an autonomous business operation with its own identity, business plan, and accountability for clinical, marketing, and financial performance. Leadership by a strong and competent administrator who thoroughly understands and believes in SRMC is essential for integrating SRMC within the organization's other product lines.

Although the hospital's administrator may be responsible for other services in the organization, this person will also administer SRMC as a service line and will oversee the provision of every function of the SRMC service, including clinical services, business operation, personnel, medical staff, marketing, and ancillary and support services. Depending on the size of the operation, most of these functions may be provided through others, such as a clinical director, a business manager, and a nursing manager. Other services are contracted out to the parent organization or to external resources (see Chapter 7). The point is not that SRMC should have a full-time administrator, but that there should be one person with complete authority over all the different services that are provided for SRMC by staff, the parent organization, and external resources.

Optimally, the administrator is involved in development from the beginning, working with the developer and program and facility development team to ensure the smooth transition of responsibility once the service has been opened.

DEVELOPMENT STAGE I: DEFINING THE PRODUCT

Despite the best of strategic plans, without strong leadership it is possible for a program and facility to be so ravaged by compromise during development that it will never be able to function as originally intended. Developing a program that is faithful to the strategic plan is critical in determining whether the organization's investment will pay off.

Following the Organization's Strategic Plan

Program and facility development should achieve defined objectives laid out during the organization's strategic planning. Before beginning development, the organization's strategic plans for SRMC are reviewed from a development viewpoint. Any questions or inconsistencies are resolved with the administration of the parent organization.

An SRMC operation works best if all of its components are in place and fully functional before starting. SRMC is difficult to achieve through a series of modifications to an existing multitransfer system. All components of the clinical, marketing, and business programs should be in place, and medical and nursing staff development should be at an appropriate level before the new SRMC facility is opened. Because it takes time for attitudes and practices to change, construction often begins before every person who will be practicing in the SRMC program has come to understand and accept its concepts. The developer must ensure that the facility is designed for the optimum program of SRMC, and not for a transitional stage that medical and nursing staff may be passing through. For example, a newborn nursery should not be planned because the nursing staff are not yet supportive of mother–baby nursing or have not yet been trained to provide this type of nursing care. The developer and administrator will be responsible for preparing the staff to be able to practice mother–baby nursing by the time the facility opens.

Concept Definition

The first step of concept definition is to create one or more conceptual models of the SRMC program and facility in a baseline functional program and space plan. These models must meet the SRMC program goals, and also meet the organization's strategic plan requirements. Several iterations of the program and facility model may be needed as the concept is refined—usually to conform to the organization's capital budget.

These conceptual models incorporate SRMC programs appropriate to the size and type of service proposed and include a preliminary functional and space program. In addition, site options and conceptual facility drawings are produced. Operating revenue and cost assumptions are also input to develop a pro forma contributions projection. The costs of developing the clinical program and of designing, engineering, and building the facility are estimated and are input into the financial model.

Each element of the program must be crafted to meet the program goals of SRMC. Each program and facility element must be carefully planned to gain support. Each must be protected from corruption by declared or surreptitious resistance to change. Development team members must gain support for their plans from their colleagues who will work in the new system without compromising important program or design elements. The developer is charged with making this happen. Once an acceptable concept, cost, and pro forma are produced, the approved conceptual models are formally presented to the organization for approval.

The Functional Program and Space Plan

Once approved, the facility and program models must move from concept to reality. The developer creates a functional and space plan, which is a list of functional areas within SRMC, with occupied square footage. The total is aggregated to an estimate of space required. The developer translates the functional and space plan to a conceptual space layout, conceptual program, and facility model. The planning team members test their understanding of the general needs of an SRMC program and facility and the specific needs of their organization by responding to the conceptual program and facility model. To facilitate the decision-making process, the model developed by the program and facility developer serves as a beginning point for discussion. Because the developer's conceptual model was developed in harmony with the organization's strategic plan and goals and has already received the approval of the planning team and the organization, it provides an indication of the service and financial parameters that the development team can work within.

When needed, refinement of the functional program is done in collaboration with the program and facility development team. Decisions must be made on a wide variety of issues concerning the scope, character, and needs of clinical care, of families and visitors, of community, and of staff (Figure 7-3). Furnishings, technology, and equipment being considered must also be factored into the functional program and space plan.

A good written functional program provides considerable detail about the goals to be achieved. Each function is assigned an adequate amount of space, and costs are accurately estimated. Basic relationships between functions are described. Overall expansion requirements are identified, and maximum budget allowances are clarified. A successful program will not only meet program goals related to care, it will also need to meet business goals and provide an environment that medical and nursing staff will accept and comfortably work in. The developer's challenge will be to gather and respond to input from physicians, nurses, administration, and families while preserving the integrity of the program and

facility design. This can be a problem if there is reluctance to adopt unfamiliar concepts or if the concepts are not well understood.

At this stage of program planning, the practical implications of an SRMC program design are fully recognized by medical and nursing staff, both on the maternity service and in other departments such as pediatrics and anesthesiology. There may be considerable pressure from departments and individuals to compromise the design to accommodate conventional or transitional practices. Staff may pressure the team to reorder design priorities toward a more standard model or to obtain personal or departmental advantage. In some instances, these changes could seriously compromise the function or efficiency of the SRMC program and add considerably to both capital and/or operational costs. Corruption of SRMC design principles can add millions of dollars to construction costs while resulting in facilities that do not function well.

If a powerful individual lobbies for a change in the SRMC program that would interfere with achievement of SRMC goals, the development team should be well prepared with factual justification to defend the design's functional integrity. The team must be able to count on the support of the parent organization's leadership to maintain

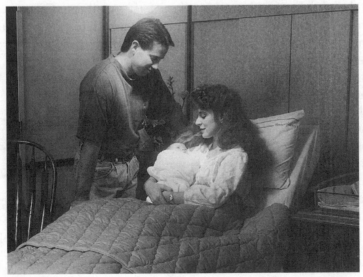

FIGURE 7–3. Families come first when planning the SRMC program and facility. (Photo courtesy of Pomona Valley Medical Center, Pomona, CA.)

consistency with the organization's strategic plan. Often, education space is the first to go when a facility project must be scaled down. In SRMC, family education takes priority, and loss of education space can compromise the SRMC program.

Review of Program Plan

The first development stage is complete when the team has reached consensus on the clinical programming, the facility functional plan, and the details of use, size, and relationship of spaces within the facility. The developer, with the assistance of the architect, clinical service leaders, and financial services, now produces a detailed clinical and functional program and detailed floor plans, site plans, and elevations of the facility, together with cost estimates for program development and implementation and for facility construction. The development team reviews this detailed operational, facility, and financial model, and then seeks approval from the parent organization.

Financial Model Development

The initial financial pro formas are developed in concert with concept definition. By the end of stage I of the development process, the program is sufficiently defined to allow the completion of a preliminary financial model. A properly designed model will permit the organization to evaluate the financial impact of various alternative strategies (often referred to as "what if" scenarios). It allows evaluation of potential changes in facility utilization, market share, case mix, payer mix, staffing, facilities investment, and any other costs associated with SRMC services and facility. This can be a complex process and generally requires the services of a specialist with experience both in financial modeling and in maternity program management. Models are generally designed for 3- or 5-year time frames.

Usually, the key outputs from the modeling process are maternity program contribution margin, net cash flow, and/or return on investment (ROI). ROI measures the projected rewards from an investment over the cost of making the investment. Financial modeling includes all of the various diagnoses that compose the clinical program.

This is particularly important when a hospital expects that its improvements in programs and services will bring in more families and/or increase contract reimbursement levels.

After completing utilization projections, costs are projected based on the organization's cost-accounting data. Some costs are variable, that is, they vary with utilization changes; others are fixed, meaning they do not depend on utilization. Initiating a new SRMC program requires new staffing patterns that will complicate cost projection, and future costs will not necessarily reflect past history. The modeler must understand the "components" of each cost category so staffing costs can be projected separately if necessary. The outcome of this process is a financial picture of the results of the program plan, business plan, and facility functional and space plans that meets the approval of the organization and its stakeholders.

Decision to Build

If program and facility are approved, construction drawings are authorized and the remaining development tasks proceed. These include development of equipment requirements, clinical and business policies and procedures, medical and nursing staff education programs, staffing program, marketing program, and recruitment of key staff members. Construction of the facility may be negotiated or put out to bid, and contracts are awarded for program implementation and for facility construction.

DEVELOPMENT STAGE II: FACILITY CONSTRUCTION AND PROGRAM IMPLEMENTATION

Building healthcare facilities is a specialized process. Building a new type of healthcare facility such as an SRMC facility requires an additional level of understanding of special design, engineering, construction, interior design, and equipment requirements. In the case of SRMC, many design and construction principles are different from those found anywhere else in an acute-care hospital. To ensure that construction conforms to program requirements, it is important for the developer to function as "owner's representative," controlling or closely monitoring construction and equipping of the new facility.

Construction Oversight

Proper management of the construction or renovation project will help to ensure that the SRMC program is able to accomplish its mission in a facility that is functional, efficient, and aesthetically pleasing. The developer serves as the owner's representative during the construction phase, and oversees the general contractor or construction manager to ensure that the organization achieves the facility that it specifies, and that the project is completed on time and within budget. Control over the process is maintained through weekly meetings during which construction progress, problems, and corrective actions are discussed. Chaired by the developer, the meeting includes the architect, general contractor or construction manager, subcontractors, and such members of the organization management team as may be appropriate for that week's agenda items. The meeting should be held faithfully each week, based on a written agenda, and documented.

Another key role for the developer during the construction or renovation phase is regular inspections of all aspects of the work. The inspections should be at irregular times and should involve observation, listening, and recording of issues to be resolved at the weekly project meetings. Change orders are a fact of life during a construction or renovation project. They may occur because of unforeseen construction or engineering problems, or they may simply reflect the continuing evolution of planning for the new program. In any event, the developer ensures that an up-to-date estimate of project costs, including change orders, is made so that appropriate reporting can be made to the organization relative to project budget status.

Program Implementation

While construction of the facility takes place, all remaining aspects of SRMC program development must be completed and its infrastructure put in place. Equipment and furnishings must be selected and purchased. Services such as food service, housekeeping, and communications must be arranged. Relationships must be formalized with both internal (hospital) and external resources. Nursing and other staff must be educated. Clinical, administrative, and business policies must be developed and adopted. Provider practices must be developed to support the SRMC model of care. The marketing program must be developed for implementation before the service opens.

During this process, careful attention is paid to gaining support for the new service. Well-established cultures are very resistant to change. Changing ingrained practices can violate cultural mores and beliefs and may be perceived as threats, even as a personal attack. Unless everyone involved buys into the new model, staff will not make changes even if they are unhappy with the status quo. However, they can be inspired or motivated to do so.

Effective change requires building on the existing culture (O'Toole, 1995). Every organization, including a hospital, has a unique system of values, beliefs, and behaviors that exert a powerful and pervasive influence on how the organization operates, but those who participate in it are not consciously aware of it. They simply believe that theirs is the only right and proper way of doing things (Gerteis, Levitan-Edgman, Daley & Delbanco, 1993).

This has important consequences for introducing a new program into a traditional maternity service. The traditional hospital maternity service is divided into distinct territories: labor and delivery, postpartum, and nursery. Physical boundaries are usually strictly observed, and staff members within each subspecialty often develop a certain clannishness. Staff members in one maternity area may have little understanding or appreciation of the work done in other areas and a distrust of blurring boundaries between areas. So, for example, postpartum staff may refer to labor and delivery as "the back," or nursery nurses may think that babies are only safe in the nursery. Staff members who cross boundaries, such as, for example, the postpartum nurse who offers to help out in labor and delivery on a busy day, may face resentment, and her services may be discounted by both medical and nursing staffs.

The divisions can also foster unhealthy competition. Struggles for power can occur between the separate units and their separate managers or between different clinical departments such as OB/GYN and pediatrics or anesthesia. This bodes ill for SRMC, which requires cooperation between subspecialties and integration of care. Such power struggles have the potential to be damaging to families as well as staff.

People who choose a career in health care usually do so because they want to help others. For this reason, once they understand the benefits of an SRMC program for childbearing families, they may be willing to tolerate the discomfort of change. Sometimes, recognition of the maternity service's weakening competitive position, declining financial performance, family dissatisfaction, or emerging competition can facilitate the sense of urgency that will motivate change.

No culture change happens easily or quickly. It may take a considerable length of time to convert a traditional hospital-focused culture to a family-focused culture and an SRMC program. However, patience and persistence will be rewarded, provided that those who hope to induce change recognize the importance of cultural inertia and are prepared to address it. With success, the new philosophy will become part of the fabric of the organization.

Nursing Staff Development

The most important factor in successfully implementing family-centered maternity care is a change in staff attitudes and practice (Minister of Supply and Services Canada, 1987). Although health care professionals and families have similar needs and goals for the childbirth experience, the emphasis may be different. Although both want a healthy baby and mother and a positive experience, parents concern themselves more with the quality of the birth experience than medical staff and nursing staff tend to do. Interestingly, however, what makes for a more positive experience—informed choice, limited intervention, sensitive and supportive care, not being sep-

arated from the baby—also makes for a healthier mother and baby and a stronger family (Bryanton, Fraser-Davey & Sullivan, 1994; Hodnett, 1996; Korte & Scaer, 1992; Simkin, 1986; Tarka & Paunonen, 1996).

Change

Although SRMC can produce dramatic improvements in patient and staff satisfaction, not all staff will find it easy to embrace the new model. All change, by definition, is unsettling to some degree. Some nursing staff will be uncomfortable with their new roles and increased autonomy. Staff can be helped to make the transition by a formal change management program. The emphasis is on the nature of the changes and how the changes will benefit staff personally and professionally as well as the families they serve. It helps staff deal with their feelings about the change. Attention to these issues and concerns allows each person to adapt more productively. Nonetheless, some nursing staff turnover may be inevitable.

Attitude Surveys

Before developing a nursing staff change program, staff is surveyed to elicit feelings and concerns about the new program. These issues are then addressed during the change process. A survey instrument that assesses the attitudes of maternity nursing staff regarding family-centered maternity care practices can be used (Phillips & Fenwick, 1992). The survey analysis frequently reveals erroneous beliefs about care that must be changed or they will impede the successful achievement of family-centered care.

For example, if nurses believe that "safety" equates with confinement to bed in labor, routine IVs, and continuous electronic fetal monitoring, they will not be receptive to, and may not follow, policies and procedures that state that laboring women may be ambulatory and have intermittent fetal monitoring. If, however, they can be led to understand that normal labor does not require such interventions, they will be open to implementing family-centered maternity care practices and policies because doing so no longer compromises their beliefs about what constitutes safe care.

Change Workshops

It may be tempting to ignore or deny staff attitudes because it can be painful and difficult to acknowledge and deal with them; however, not doing so can result in even more pain and difficulty and the possibility that the change process may fail (Moore & Komras, 1993).

A survey of staff attitudes toward family-centered care precedes workshops to help staff cope with the changeover to SRMC. Workshops disseminate a vision of change, educate staff members about the new care models, and encourage them to express their feelings about the change. Change workshops provide a context for airing legitimate professional concerns and enable staff to participate in the change process. Staff are taught positive verbal and nonverbal communication strategies and ways of dealing with conflict that can be used in dealing with coworkers in the professional setting or with family and friends in personal life.

Change workshops result in staff better understanding the SRMC program and also being better prepared to make the transition. Because it is important that everyone receives the same information and has the opportunity to have his or her concerns addressed, attendance at change workshops is mandatory. The workshop also may help some staff members to realize that they cannot or do not want to change, and these individuals can be transferred to another position in the organization if appropriate.

Physicians

For an SRMC program to work in harmony, and for the family-oriented goals of the program to be met, all providers must support the service's philosophy of care and practice according to its principles of care. The key to developing and maintaining consistent and appropriate professional practice is the appointment of a clinical director, who is responsible for assessing, training, and monitoring medical and nursing practice on the SRMC service. SRMC practice is encouraged and monitored by integrating evidence-based practice parameters into all regular professional forums, such as the SRMC departmental meeting, journal club meetings, and various clinical meetings. Participation in the clinical development program described in Chapter 3 is made a condition for practicing in the unit, as is continued demonstration of practices that support the mission and goals of the service.

Marketing

Although the development of the marketing program may be contracted out to the parent organization or to an external resource, it remains the responsibility of the administrator. The marketing program must reflect SRMC's unique positioning and marketing goals and also should tie in to the hospital's overall marketing goals. Marketing strategy is based on research information and the maternity service's positioning objectives. Marketing goals and objectives for the SRMC service should be established and used to measure progress after implementation.

A marketing plan includes communication strategies that educate families about the benefits of family-centered care and builds pride among groups who can identify with the hospital. The strategic marketing plan should include carefully constructed messages to reach target audiences. The plan should have defined and measurable targets and advertising and promotional tactics to achieve desired positioning. The plan should be formally adopted with timelines for implementation based on the unit's opening. Marketing will be discussed in detail in Chapter 8.

Family Education Services

Comprehensive educational programs are developed for various inpatient programs. These programs may be provided as private education or in small groups. Generally, these programs are taught by the most experienced educators because of the need for the educator to rapidly assess and respond to the individual families encountered. The educator may make rounds to antepartum, postpartum, NICU units, or may respond to a physician or CNM order for educational services or both.

Community Education Programming

The childbirth education program not only complements but also is an integral component of an SRMC program. A number of factors influence the integration of childbirth education into clinical service. Organizationally, the childbirth education program is placed within the structure of maternal/newborn services. When programs are placed in marketing, education, or support services, this dissociates the program in multiple ways.

Both the program manager's office and some classroom space are located on or adjacent to the SRMC facility. Physical distance dissociates the program from practice. Further, integrated programs serve a high volume of inpatient families. This is more likely if a phone call requesting services is made to an office down the hall rather than down the street or across town. Education rounds are more easily managed from this close proximity as well.

The childbirth education program reflects the full scope of outpatient and inpatient clinical practice. The program developed for a level one hospital or freestanding birth center staffed by midwives will look different than a program designed for a tertiary-care center that has a high-risk antepartum unit and a NICU. The program developed reflects the range of families served by the organization. An organization that has a large teen population or poor families who may find transportation a challenge and child care a barrier to class participation will design a different program than one located in the suburbs with a largely middle-income population with two working parents.

Integration is enhanced when at least 50% of the childbirth education program staff is maternity staff working a portion of the time in the SRMC program. These staff should, of course, be certified childbirth educators.

Orientation of all new SRMC employees includes an introduction to components of the childbirth education program. Also included are waived or reduced fees for all childbirth education program services as part of the benefits package for hospital employees, thus increasing the link between their work and this program.

Programmatic Approach

In SRMC programs, childbirth education services are designed from a programmatic approach rather than viewed as classes that function independently of one another. Through integration strategies, the program reflects the philosophy of family-centered care and the clinical scope of practice. However, internal integration is equally important. Such internal integration creates a seamless educational approach that allows families to make a connection to the program even before pregnancy and continue well into the first year postpartum with a sense of educational continuity that supports their work in the unfolding process of family development. Methods of developing internal integration follow.

An educational vision retreat is held for all educators and key stakeholders in clinical practice to look at the process of childbearing from preconception through the first year postpartum. Critical touch points for education are identified, and a framework for program development that reflects those touch points is created. Next, the touch points are made seamless so that as families move through the educational program, the program builds on educational experiences—filling in gaps and/or acknowledging where families have already been. The vision retreat also explores strategies for development or improvement of curriculum. Methods of ensuring that all who have contact with the childbearing family understand the educational program—both in terms of the whole and parts—should also be described. Providing families with a personal education guidebook that reflects a vision created for educational wellness through the childbearing year invites them to view the process as one of growth rather than discrete experiences.

Curricula are designed and reviewed annually for characteristics of internal as well as scope of practice integration. Hiring, staff orientation, and staff development of employees of the childbirth education program are continually directed toward maintaining a staff that understands the vision and full scope of education services and the goal of SRMC. Childbirth education program staff meetings are held on at least a quarterly basis with all educators in attendance. These quarterly meetings may include reports from work groups that are involved in continued program growth or development. A primary objective of the quarterly meeting, however, is team building and education that works to sustain the vision of integrated services.

Contracted Services

Maternity services operate around the clock, and it is essential that time-sensitive services providing support to SRMC be likewise available. Whether professional and support services are provided directly by the SRMC program or are contracted through the parent or other organizations, they should always be responsible to the SRMC administrator. Only in this way can the SRMC administrator ensure consistency of quality and ensure that all professional and support services staff understand and support the SRMC philosophy.

Services that often are contracted through a parent or independent organization include medical records, transcription, coding, credentialing, human resources (recruitment and benefits administration in particular), information systems support, communications (telephone systems), nutrition services, laboratory, blood bank, EKG, respiratory therapy, maintenance, clinical engineering, purchasing, and accreditation/licensure support. Services are enumerated in written contracts where possible. The SRMC administrator is ultimately responsible for all that occurs in the program, and the contract documents should spell out very clearly the role of the contractor and the role of the SRMC program as customer.

Services contracted through external sources obviously require written contracts. Externally contracted services often include housekeeping, linen and laundry, medical and business information systems, grounds maintenance (if appropriate), and security.

Of course, these lists are not intended to be exhaustive—some services listed as potential external contracts may be purchased from the parent hospital and vice versa. In addition, some services listed may be available through a management contractor. However, the need for autonomy of the SRMC program and comprehensive authority of the SRMC administrator remains constant. All contracts, with whatever source, must be under the control of the administrator.

The Business Plan

Once adopted, this is a formal strategic business plan to guide business strategy, program development, provider practice acquisition, contract negotiation, and marketing decisions for SRMC. This plan is designed from a strategic perspective and is driven by an assessment of the family health, maternity, and newborn needs of the community. It defines the comprehensive care of the childbearing family, illustrates strong financial performance, and describes a comprehensive marketing strategy for the program.

Strategic Objectives

The last component of the business plan is the development of objectives, and specific actions whose accomplishment will achieve organizational goals. Objectives describe what an organization wants to occur to achieve the identified goals. They state what will constitute success in observable and measurable terms, and have a specified time horizon. Strategic objectives should contain specific benchmarking targets so progress can be measured. Box 7-1 is a listing of some sample categories for which strategic objectives are developed.

QUALITY IMPROVEMENT AND PROGRAM EVALUATION

Comprehensive quality management programs do more than just measure performance. In successful SRMC programs, effective quality

B O X   7 – 1

Sample Categories for Which Strategic Objectives Are Developed

MARKETING TARGETS

- Hospital market share
- Market share of maternity services

FINANCIAL TARGETS

- Maternity contribution margin
- Payer mix
- Collection percentages
- Revenue/expense ratios
- Budget variances
- Days of revenue in accounts receivable
- FTEs per occupied bed or patient day

CLINICAL TARGETS

- Number of births
- Cesarean rate
- VBAC rate
- Induction rate
- Nursing hours per case

improvement programs make the organization's vision happen. Effective quality management programs focus the efforts of people throughout the organization toward achieving strategic objectives. These programs also provide feedback about current performance and help establish realistic targets for future performance.

The successful implementation of a quality management program within an organization can have a dramatic impact in a number of areas. Although many companies rely on performance measurement systems that incorporate financial and nonfinancial measures, these are often only used for control and feedback of short-term operations at a corporate level.

Measuring the success of the organization's business strategy through financial monitoring can reveal areas in which improvement is needed. Monitoring provider performance through benchmarking can provide information about how individual providers perform in relationship

with providers practicing in similar organizations. This gives the use of performance measures a broader perspective and gives a measure of "best practice." Operationally, the organization can monitor improvements in communication, teambuilding, and strategic priority setting as related to implementation of the SRMC program. Customer satisfaction measures allow the organization to monitor the success of the SRMC program in attracting customers from target groups such as key neighborhoods, select managed care contracts, and so forth. In addition, measuring customer satisfaction with specific program components can allow the organization to measure its success in implementing family-centered practices and programs that are attractive to young families.

Measuring Success Using Benchmarking

The SRMC program can implement a benchmarking process using internal data and measuring that data against externally published outcomes data. Benchmarking is a means of comparing one organization or person to a better performer (or the best) and learning why the poorer performer is not as good (Goldfield, 1999). This might mean looking at best practices in cost reduction in another industry and identifying how to apply these to the maternity service. Best practices are defined as those practices and processes that support and enhance the outcomes of an organization and represent sound clinical, operational, and financial performance (Fitzgerald, 1998).

Sometimes, identification of appropriate benchmarks is difficult for an individual hospital or SRMC program. In the event a management company is involved, the SRMC administrator should expect the management company to have access to benchmarks and to provide useful feedback about the SRMC program's comparison to similar programs.

Patient Satisfaction Surveys

Quality of service, or the manner in which patient care is delivered, is typically measured by patient satisfaction surveys.

It is important to collect consumer feedback only when it becomes possible for the woman to discriminate between the happy experience of the birth of a healthy baby and the care she actually received. Questionnaires given to women still in the hospital will not provide valid answers because of the halo effect. In the mother's mind, the birth of a healthy baby may help compensate for any negative experiences.

The organization can mail a written consumer satisfaction questionnaire to families after discharge. The questionnaire includes instructions to fill out the form and return it to the hospital (either a postage-paid self-mailer can be used or a stamped envelope addressed to the hospital can be included in the questionnaire). Some hospitals distribute such a questionnaire at the time of discharge; however, it may be mislaid in the preparations to go home.

If the hospital already uses a general consumer satisfaction questionnaire, it may wish to incorporate maternity service questions in the general form or include an extra page for maternity patients. General questions about the quality of nursing care will not provide specific feedback about the aspects of family-centered care.

For example, nursing managers need to know if mothers feel comfortable feeding their babies at discharge, if they had their baby with them as much as desired, and if their questions were answered satisfactorily. Of additional value is space for comments.

Questionnaire design is a highly developed skill. Special care must be taken not to ask leading questions. Development of a questionnaire can be jointly undertaken by clinicians with primary support provided by marketing staff, by the management contractor, or by professional consumer researchers.

Once a questionnaire has been developed and tested and a distribution mechanism determined, the compilation and review process should be established. If computer entry of questionnaire data is to be made, the form should be designed with this fact in mind. Questionnaire results and comments must be summarized frequently and presented to medical and nursing staffs for review and discussion.

Making it easy for consumers to express their opinions increases the probability that comments will be made. Many hospitals have mechanisms such as a 24-hour "hot line" for consumer comment. Exit interviews of women before discharge is another way of listening.

Quality management programs emphasize the importance of using financial and nonfinancial measures to inform employees about progress and success at all levels of the organization. When the organization plans and integrates a focus on quality into all aspects of an SRMC program, it will experience success in terms of finances, provider practice, operational targets, and customer satisfaction. All of these areas are equally critical to the long-term success of the SRMC program.

SUMMARY

Implementing change within an organization is fraught with pitfalls. Strategic planning and a structured development process help to avoid those pitfalls by developing initial parameters within which planning and development take place. In addition, a well-designed SRMC development process can foster cooperation and enthusiasm for the new program by including representatives of all the stakeholder groups in the project implementation.

REFERENCES

Bryanton, J., Fraser-Davey, H., & Sullivan, P. (1994). Women's perceptions of nursing support during labor. *Journal of Obstetric, Gynecologic, and Neonatal Nursing, 23*(8), 638–644.

Fitzgerald, K. (1998). Clinical benchmarking: Implications for perinatal nursing. *Journal of Perinatal Neonatal Nursing, 12*(1), 23–30.

Gerteis, J., Levitan-Edgman, S., Daley, J., & Delbanco, T. L., (Eds.). (1993). *Through the patient's eyes: Understanding and promoting patient-centered care.* San Francisco: Jossey-Bass.

Goldfield, N. (1999). *Physician profiling and risk adjustment* (2nd ed.). Gaithersburg, MD: Aspen.

Hodnett, E. (1996). Nursing support of the laboring woman. *Journal of Obstetric, Gynecologic, and Neonatal Nursing, 25*(3), 257–264.

Korte, D., & Scaer, R. (1992). *A good birth, a safe birth* (3rd rev. ed.). Boston: Harvard Common Press.

Minister of Supply and Services Canada. (1987). *Family-centered maternity and newborn care: National guidelines*. Ottawa, Canada: Ministry of National Health and Welfare.

Moore, N., & Komras, H. (1993). *Patient-focused healing: Integrating caring and curing in health care*. San Francisco: Jossey-Bass.

O'Toole, J. (1995). *Leading change: Overcoming the ideology of comfort and the tyranny of custom*. San Francisco: Jossey-Bass.

Phillips, C. R., & Fenwick, L. (1992). *Phillips+Fenwick nurse attitude survey instrument*. Unpublished.

Simkin, P. (1986). Stress, pain, and catecholamines in labor: Part 2. Stress associated with childbirth events: A pilot survey of new mothers. *Birth, 13*(4), 234–240.

Tarka, M. T., & Paunonen, M. (1996). Social support and its impact on mothers' experiences of childbirth. *Journal of Advanced Nursing, 23*(1), 70–75.

Trofino, J. (1995, August). Transformational leadership in health care. *Nursing Management, 26*(8), 42–47.

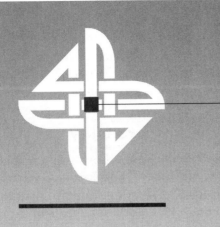

CHAPTER 8

Single-Room Maternity Care Operations

For decades, organizations have found it advantageous for certain specialized clinical services to operate with a large measure of autonomy. In many hospitals, radiology, laboratory, and emergency care services operate as separate business units. One reason for this arrangement is that specialized services need skills and flexibility to develop and operate these programs that may not be available in a typical acute-care hospital. Another reason is to keep these services aligned with the hospital to avoid the risk of their being established externally in competition with the hospital.

In recent years, clinical services such as cardiology and radiology have begun to shift out of the acute-care hospital facility into separate facilities. Away from the cultural and bureaucratic restraints of a large organization, these facilities and programs have, in some instances, developed exemplary services that have quickly gained market share and become highly profitable.

THE CORE BUSINESS MODEL

Traditionally, hospitals have operated maternity departments in much the same way that they have operated other acute-care services such as medical, surgical, or pediatric services. It is possible for hospitals to merely upgrade their conventional maternity departments and continue to operate them as they do other acute-care services. However, an SRMC program needs a fresh start to break the bonds of old services and old thinking, and then needs to have a large measure of control over all care and other activities provided on the service in order to maintain the character, quality, and consistency of its service. When a business model is largely self-sufficient and independent of its parent organization, it is known as a core business model.

SRMC represents a reengineered system of delivering OB services—from the clinical practice to the facility design. The scope of care is different in SRMC programs, requiring the hospital to assume responsibility for the operation of education and support programs as well as inpatient services provided for labor and birth. SRMC programs can create and project a family-friendly image to the community and provide new positioning for the entire organization. If a maternity program is to play a new role in its relationship to the community and the overall hospital, it will require a different management approach. To allow it to develop and maintain its unique operations and character, an administrator committed to the integrity and success of the SRMC program coordinates every aspect of care.

SRMC LEADERSHIP

The administrator develops, organizes, and manages every aspect of the project and is given the support, budget, and authority necessary to achieve success. The right person for this important role will have a thorough understanding of the organization's strategic plan and will understand how to operationalize that plan in the SRMC program. This administrator must have the ability to manage the service at a high level of safety, satisfaction, and efficiency so the organization as a whole benefits from the SRMC program's success.

The Administrator

For the remainder of this chapter, the term *administrator* will be used to signify the administrative function, whether filled by an individual employed by the organization or contracted through a women's healthcare company. If the administrator is a hospital employee, he or she will usually have responsibility for additional hospital services. If the administrator is an employee of a women's healthcare company, he or she may administer other services as well.

The administrator reports directly to the parent organization's chief executive officer (CEO) and directs all business, medical, nursing, marketing, and management functions of the SRMC service. The administrator needs the support of the parent hospital, its management team, clinical staff, and physician leadership, and that of various community leaders to ensure the program's success.

The administrator is responsible for business plan development and may be responsible for contracting with payers if this is done separately from the parent organization. Once the facility development process is complete, the administrator will assume responsibility for its operation, for the program's financial performance, for the management of all SRMC business operations and clinical care programs, and for communicating the SRMC program's image and message to the parent organization and the community. Control of marketing messages, both externally and internally, and assurance of quality management and risk management programs are part of the administrator's responsibilities.

Flow of Responsibility

Figure 8-1 illustrates how the administrator is responsible for all business operations, clinical operations, ancillary and support operations, and marketing. This does not mean that the SRMC service should have its own administrator whose only responsibility is SRMC! Instead, it means that SRMC should be under the authority of only one administrator, so that operations in SRMC are not controlled by a variety of managers responsible for other hospital services provided in SRMC. It is particularly important that SRMC have a strong champion who understands the needs of the program and who can ensure that the SRMC service has the latitude to select personnel and services necessary for its program of care.

The administrator responsible for SRMC has overall authority of operations of the SRMC unit. Depending on the size of the SRMC unit, each of these operations could be managed by one or more managers who report to the administrator. Thus, in a women's specialty hospital where SRMC is provided along with other women's services, the hospital would have its own administrator who would direct a business manager, a clinical director, one or more nurse managers, and a marketing manager. In women's centers where SRMC is provided along with women's ambulatory and diagnostic healthcare services, this administrator would have service line responsibility over SRMC, women's services, and other departments. In hospitals with SRMC units not associated with other women's services, the administrator would be shared with other hospital departments.

Another option is to outsource administration and management of SRMC. In this situation, the SRMC manager may report to an outside company that, in turn, reports to the parent hospital CEO. Whether the administrator is on the management company's staff or not, the important issue is that all operations of SRMC be under consistent control to maintain the safety, satisfac-

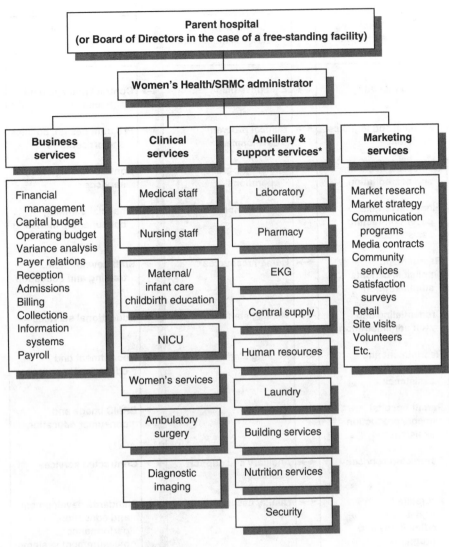

Parent hospital
(or Board of Directors in the case of a free-standing facility)

Women's Health/SRMC administrator

Business services	Clinical services	Ancillary & support services*	Marketing services
Financial management Capital budget Operating budget Variance analysis Payer relations Reception Admissions Billing Collections Information systems Payroll	Medical staff Nursing staff Maternal/ infant care childbirth education NICU Women's services Ambulatory surgery Diagnostic imaging	Laboratory Pharmacy EKG Central supply Human resources Laundry Building services Nutrition services Security	Market research Market strategy Communication programs Media contracts Community services Satisfaction surveys Retail Site visits Volunteers Etc.

FIGURE 8–1. Service organization chart. The administrator reports to the parent organization CEO and is directly responsible for all aspects of SRMC operation.

* Administrator's authority is limited to components of these services that are provided to Women's Health/SRMC

tion, efficiency, and program integrity of the SRMC service.

Resources Available to Support SRMC Operations

Figure 8-2 shows how the administrator uses internal and external resources to obtain and control all the elements necessary for the operation of the SRMC program and facility. Some services needed for operation of the service may be contracted from the parent organization, and others may be contracted through external sources. Whatever combination of resources that the administrator uses to operate the SRMC service, all operations performed in the SRMC program are under the direction of the SRMC administrator.

There must be a close working relationship between the CEO of the parent hospital and the administrator responsible for SRMC. The administrator must be able to keep the program on track as it develops and matures, while ensuring that the parent hospital's mission and policy direction are faithfully followed.

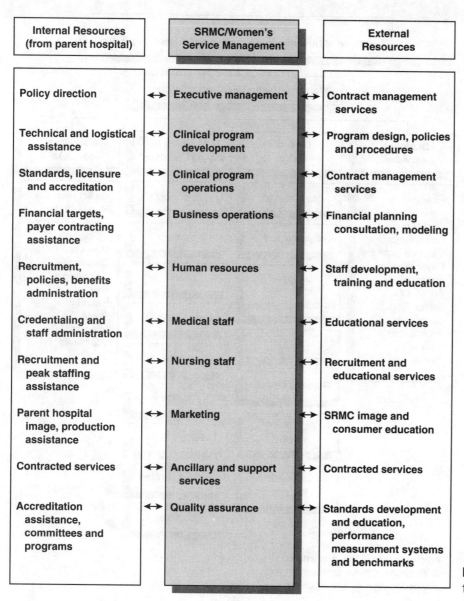

Internal Resources (from parent hospital)	SRMC/Women's Service Management	External Resources
Policy direction	↔ Executive management ↔	Contract management services
Technical and logistical assistance	↔ Clinical program development ↔	Program design, policies and procedures
Standards, licensure and accreditation	↔ Clinical program operations ↔	Contract management services
Financial targets, payer contracting assistance	↔ Business operations ↔	Financial planning consultation, modeling
Recruitment, policies, benefits administration	↔ Human resources ↔	Staff development, training and education
Credentialing and staff administration	↔ Medical staff ↔	Educational services
Recruitment and peak staffing assistance	↔ Nursing staff ↔	Recruitment and educational services
Parent hospital image, production assistance	↔ Marketing ↔	SRMC image and consumer education
Contracted services	↔ Ancillary and support services ↔	Contracted services
Accreditation assistance, committees and programs	↔ Quality assurance ↔	Standards development and education, performance measurement systems and benchmarks

FIGURE 8–2. SRMC operations—resource management.

To succeed as a core business enterprise, the SRMC program must have a high level of autonomy, particularly in the selection of leadership staff. Individuals selected to manage critical functions must understand the unique nature of SRMC programs and must have special skills in operationalizing programs.

BUSINESS OPERATIONS

The language of business is accounting, and that means it is necessary for the SRMC program to be able to demonstrate its financial results in terms that are accurate, clear, and concise.

Financial Management

The administrator must have in place a financial management structure that involves at least three components—budgeting, financial reporting, and variance analysis. Although these three components will generally be governed by the guidelines of the parent organization, it is important that the administrator of the SRMC understands each component and actively participates in the business management process.

The budget is nothing more than a plan for the financial operation of the business enterprise for some future period of time. Usually the budget is prepared for the hospital's fiscal year—often different from the calendar year. The fiscal year is determined by an organization's governing board and represents the normal annual operating cycle for the business. Budgets for a fiscal year will generally also include monthly breakdowns to assist in comparing actual results each month to budgeted amounts.

Budgets often include two distinct components—capital budgets and operating budgets. The capital budget covers those planned purchases that are generally referred to as property and equipment. Capital budget items usually have a useful life of more than 1 year, and the cost of capital purchases is not charged directly to the operation of a business entity when the purchase is made. Instead, the anticipated useful life of the property or equipment is estimated, and the cost of the purchase is then spread throughout the useful life through an expense item called depreciation.

The operating budget covers those revenues and costs generated by, or expended in, the day-to-day operation of the business enterprise. In the SRMC program, the operating budget will generally include revenues from services to patients, staffing costs (including payroll taxes and benefits), drugs and supplies costs, purchased professional services (such as laboratory and radiology), and other costs such as staff education, travel, nutritional supplies, and so forth. The SRMC administrator is the key participant in developing the operating budget, using historical information and business plans for the coming fiscal year. Only by taking an active role in the development of the operating budget can the administrator ensure that the financial standards to which she or he is being held are reasonable and attainable.

The financial reporting process in most hospitals is based on a monthly summary of the revenues generated by and costs incurred by each business unit. Business units in hospitals may be referred to as cost centers, departments, business lines, or business enterprises. The hospital's finance department prepares at the close of each calendar month a report that provides the department manager with the actual results for the month, often with a comparison to budget and to the same month in the prior year. To properly evaluate these reports, the administrator must understand exactly what has been included and why. For that reason, many hospital financial managers provide supporting information to the department managers showing actual expenditures made and dates incurred. In the event this information is not routinely supplied, the SRMC administrator develops a close enough level of communication with the hospital's financial manager to obtain this information whenever needed to provide clarity to the reports.

The final, and most important, step in the business management cycle for the SRMC program is the analysis of variances between the actual financial results each month and the amounts budgeted. Most hospitals require department managers to provide written explanations for variances above a preset amount or percentage. However, whether required or not, the administrator should perform such an analysis every month, identifying reasons for variances and especially noting financial and variance trends. By maintaining constant vigilance over the financial results, the administrator can be prepared to successfully lobby for additional resources for the SRMC program as they are identified. Hospital administrators, financial managers, and board members almost invariably are more receptive to resource requests that are well documented and that are presented by program administrators who demonstrate a clear understanding of the financial management cycle.

Admissions and Business Office

The business office functions are often described by using the first three letters of the alphabet—ABC—for admissions, billing, and collections. The administrator ensures that all three of these functions are working properly and that the procedures in place are supportive of the philosophy of family-centered care. Regardless of how the services are provided, through internal staff or contract, the administrator takes an active role in managing the functions.

The admissions process is generally completed before admission. There should not be a need for the woman or her family to be detained at the "front desk" when she arrives in labor. Admission forms are completed and any necessary insurance approvals obtained before admission. In any event, all face-to-face business contacts with the woman or her family should take place in a private, nonthreatening environment.

The billing process begins during the woman's inpatient stay. During this time, any necessary contacts are made with her payer. It continues through discharge and until the time a final and complete billing is sent to the responsible insurance company or family. Generally, with proper preadmission counseling and clear understanding of financial requirements, it is not necessary for families to "check out" through the business office when they are ready to leave the facility and go home.

The collection process involves primarily the function of insurance follow-up, which represents the single most important area for ensuring the hospital's prompt recovery of amounts due for patient services. By aggressively pursuing all insurance claims and promptly responding to the inevitable requests for supporting information, the hospital can minimize the amount of its resources that are tied up in accounts receivable. Individual account collection should be minimal because payment arrangements should always be made clear with the woman and her family long before admission.

Medical Records

In many cases, the medical records, coding, and transcription functions may be contracted from the parent hospital. In any event, though, it is clear that the administrator must be actively involved in overseeing the operations so that the SRMC program's philosophy and mission are upheld. In addition, because of the frequent contact that these functions must maintain with the individual members of the SRMC professional staff, the administrator should ensure that very high standards are maintained in both verbal and written communications. In fact, the administrator may wish to require that all written communications with physicians bear the administrator's signature.

CLINICAL OPERATION

In SRMC, instead of compartmentalizing care into maternal, newborn, and NICU areas, these are integrated into an approach that focuses on continuity of care. This requires commitment to a common set of operational goals. SRMC requires that every professional practitioner support and practice according to the same set of strategic goals, a uniform set of policies and procedures, and according to the same mission.

Clinical Program Leadership

Ideally, a clinical director, who is a physician contracted to provide this service, oversees the entire program and everyone who provides care to childbearing women and families. This clinical director should be responsible for all clinical services provided by the medical and nursing staffs, including medical care, midwifery care, nursing care, and newborn intensive care. The clinical director should also be responsible for overseeing other clinical programs and operations that are provided, such as anesthesia, diagnostic services, and the educational program.

Human Resources

The success of SRMC programs depends on the recruitment of medical, nursing, and other staff who believe in and will actively support the fundamental goals of the program. Recruiting the best providers and staff ensures a sustained level of excellence in clinical services and administration. Human resources costs (wages and benefits) typically exceed 50% of a hospital's operating budget (Blancett & Flarey, 1995). As the largest single group of employees, nurses represent the largest single expenditure in the human resources budget. This is one reason that SRMC programs must conduct nursing staff recruitment and selection very carefully. The administrator must be able to recruit and select quality staff members who are committed to practicing in accord with the principles of family-centered maternity care. To do this, the parent organization's human resources department must recognize and support the administrator's authority to direct staff hiring, training, and discipline.

Medical Staff

The clinical director is responsible for medical staff education, evaluation, and credentialing (possibly through the parent hospital) to participate in the SRMC program. This applies to obstetricians, pediatricians, and family physicians as well as to anesthesiologists and nurse-midwives.

Nursing Staff

The clinical director is also ultimately responsible for nursing education, evaluation, and employment in SRMC. A clinical nurse manager may manage these functions and report to the clinical director. Because nurses deliver most patient care, the clinical nurse leader is pivotal to the successful implementation of the SRMC program. Effective nursing leadership requires very special qualities. The nurse leader's authority does not derive from the old-style autocratic model but rather through inspiring others with his or her personal vision and commitment to the values and philosophy of SRMC as exemplified through day-to-day actions and behaviors (Goleman, 1998; O'Toole, 1995). The effective nurse leader's authority derives from ability to influence the behavior of others, whatever their position in the organization (Loveridge & Cummings, 1996).

To accomplish this, the nurse leader must be committed to the goals of the SRMC program. This individual must be knowledgeable about the clinical care of childbearing women and infants and must be able to earn the respect of the medical and nursing staffs. He or she must be committed to the changes desired by the organization (Bond & Fiedler, 1999) and must have the skills to work with others to translate the vision and values of SRMC into the policies, procedures, protocols, and every-day operations (Senge, 1990).

Primary Caregiver

In SRMC, the registered nurse (RN) is the primary caregiver and functions as a liaison to other caregivers. The RN role requires a decreased emphasis on tasks and an advanced level of clinical and management skills at the bedside, which results in an increase in intellectual activities and professional accountability. Clinical care emphasizes patient education, family involvement, informed decision making, and limited intervention in the birth process. This care model results in greater continuity of care, which is tailored more specifically to the needs of individual women and their families.

SRMC Nursing Model

The SRMC model permits flexibility and efficiency of care. SRMC requires one cross-trained staff member and one manager. For this reason, the SRMC model has the potential to reduce both direct and indirect costs (Phillips, 1988; Schmid & Gerlach, 1986). When RNs are educated to provide care for laboring and birthing mothers as well as postpartum mothers and babies, they can provide mother-and-baby care or labor-and-delivery care during times of peak demand. In this way, the nursing staff functions almost as their own "on-call" pool during peaks and valleys in census. SRMC also realizes cost savings because there are no transfers except to special care nurseries. Transfer time and housekeeping time are reduced to a minimum.

Nurse Facilitator Role

In larger units, a flexibly prepared nurse facilitator (RN) is assigned for every shift. Rather than managing a preassigned patient load, this nurse facilitates care, arranges for staffing, and supervises personnel and patient flow. Instead of making decisions about the care of individual patients, the nurse facilitator acts as a problem-solver, teacher, and resource for the unit. As needed, this nurse assists and facilitates the nurses providing bedside care. It is possible that this nurse may care directly for patients as the census fluctuates, but also he or she continues to coordinate the unit staff activities. Staff nurses maintain autonomy, determining when to call the physician or midwife, contacting ancillary services on their own, and informing the nurse facilitator of their actions.

Down-Substitution

In an effort to control costs during the past decade, hospitals have scrutinized the use of human resources (Blancett & Flarey, 1995; Flarey, 1995; Hines, Smeltzer & Galletti, 1994; Krapohl & Larson, 1996; Loveridge & Cummings, 1996). Ideally, nursing tasks should be distributed according to skills. This makes the most efficient use of professional nurses' (RN) time, reduces the number of RNs needed, and permits substitution of less intensively trained caregivers (Kovner & Gergen, 1998).

Professional nurses perform numerous tasks that could be delegated to less skilled people (Pischke-Winn & Minnick, 1996). These tasks include setting up for delivery; cleaning rooms after delivery; washing infant cribs; delivering and collecting food trays; delivering ice water; cleaning instruments; conducting inventories and replenishing stock and linen; making patient beds; delivering specimens to labs; delivering prescriptions to the pharmacy; tracking test results by telephone; walking to central supply to obtain stock; clerical work; selected care tasks such as ambulation, feeding, mouth care, and bathing; and data gathering such as intake and output and vital signs.

Unlicensed Assistive Personnel (UAPs)

Unlicensed assistive personnel (UAP) are bedside healthcare workers who are not licensed. They include certified nursing assistants (CNAs) and technicians (techs) and are sometimes described as patient care extenders or partners in patient care. They support professional nursing staff, work under the direction of a registered nurse, and perform selected nursing care activities and services (Barter, McLaughlin & Thomas, 1994; Lengacher, Kent, Mabe, Heinemann & Van Cott, 1994; Lengacher, Mabe, Bowling, Heinemann, Kent & Van Cott, 1993). When utilizing UAPs,

the professional registered nurse remains the primary direct caregiver (Association of Women's Health, Obstetric and Neonatal Nurses [AWHONN], 1997).

Mini-Team

Ideally, in the SRMC nursing model one RN performs assessment, planning, intervention, and documentation for one patient. Licensed vocational nurses/licensed practical nurses (LVNs/LPNs) function at their maximum ability within the limits of the Nurse Practice Act in their particular state. This may include total patient care (under the direction of an RN) for mother–baby couplets and, in some situations, stable antepartum patients.

Properly supervised and used appropriately, UAPs and LVNs/LPNs can be a safe and cost-effective alternative to an all-professional nursing staff. In fact, if their assigned tasks do not require a full-time staff person, unit secretaries can be cross-trained to provide some level of appropriate patient care support, thereby maximizing their productivity.

Staff Mix

The ideal percentage of RN caregivers varies depending on the organization of services, human resource policies/procedures, state licensure laws, how creatively the organization looks at job functions, and the education and training of staff.

Without careful planning, attempts at reducing staffing costs can result in staffing arrangements that compromise care or in care that does not meet national standards (Irvine, Sidani & Hall, 1998; Kovner & Gergen, 1998; Krapohl & Larson, 1996). Studies conducted during the last decade suggest that professional nurse understaffing adversely affects patient outcomes (Blegen, Goode & Reed, 1998). When maternity units have a mixed staff (RNs, LPNs, UAPs), care must be taken that only professional nurses (RNs) provide nursing care, while downsubstituting non-nursing functions to UAPs; however, non-nursing duties should be performed by the lowest level practitioner available who can legally perform that task.

SRMC staffing takes into account the unique nature of maternity operations in order to achieve optimally efficient staff utilization. Specifically, planners do not simply apply ratios appropriate for medical-surgical units. Specialized patient care requirements and staff knowledge and skills demanded on an SRMC unit are considered. The importance of professional nurses and their appropriate usage in maternity care cannot be overemphasized.

Allocation of Resources

Maternity cultures seem to develop "rhythms," that is, over time, weekly activity patterns are developed. For example, physicians tend to see their high-risk patients on certain days and outpatient testing tends to be higher on those days. In allocating nurse and support staff to meet patient requirements for care, planners balance both inpatient and outpatient maternity census and acuity against the number of available, qualified nursing staff at any given time. Implementing a cost-effective SRMC program demands maximum flexibility in the use of personnel as patient census and acuity vary.

Historically, maternity care nursing needs have been based on the number of forecasted births, with additional staff allocated according to the expected percentage of cesareans (Jones, Famularo, Desta, Fulgencio & Rotondo, 1992). The system of validating the budgeted full-time equivalents (FTEs) was nursing hours per patient day (NHPPD). However, NHPPD does not take into consideration the various acuity levels found on a maternity service (Duclos-Miller, 1996). Neither forecasted births nor NHPPD is relevant for allocating nursing resources on modern-day maternity units. The variability and unpredictability of today's maternity patients require creative approaches.

Acuity System

A patient classification system (PCS) or acuity system is needed for all patients on the maternity service. Acuity is defined as the intensity of nursing resources required by a patient. It serves as an indirect measure of the severity of an illness or patient need. Classifying maternity patients as low, medium, or high risk and adding information about each patient's specific condition allow time to plan for and provide appropriate numbers and type of staff (Duclos-Miller, 1996; Freitas, Helmer & Cousins, 1987; Jones et al., 1992; Schwamb, 1989; Stenske & Ferguson, 1996).

Staffing Ratios

In planning for SRMC staffing, we use the nursing staffing ratios recommended in *Guidelines for Perinatal Care*, 4th edition (American Academy of Pediatrics [AAP] & American College of Obstetricians and Gynecologists [ACOG], 1997). These standards have gained widespread acceptance throughout maternity services.

Census-Based Scheduling

The average daily census is merely the starting point for determining staffing needs. The actual census will vary widely. For this reason, the number of personnel scheduled for any one shift should not be considered as an absolute but rather as a starting point from which actual scheduling for that shift can begin. The nurse manager, leadership team, and/or nurse facilitators look at the actual census and consider the acuity of the patient population before deciding who to call to stay home and who to tell to report for duty.

Peak Census Needs

Providing staff coverage for peak census periods requires an appropriately sized pool of flexibly available part-time and/or on-call staff who are educated in all areas of maternity care. Such a call system is either formalized, as in the application of mandatory call rotated among all staff, or informal, with the hiring of several employees who agree to be available for work on a certain schedule.

Meeting the needs of patients as well as nursing personnel while controlling costs of human resources is not easy, but it can be done. Flexible scheduling options such as on-call options, shifts that begin and end outside of the regular shift times, and part-time and call-back options can help nurses manage their personal and professional lives while allowing the SRMC program to match staffing to patient need. It is possible to be fair to people while still meeting the program needs.

Staff Performance Measurement

Performance measurement of staff satisfaction is ongoing. Position descriptions and performance appraisals clearly state that employees demonstrate the knowledge, skills, and attitudes consistent with the philosophy of family-centered care that is the foundation for SRMC. Each member on staff is held accountable for providing care that is reflective of family-centered principles. There may be times when personnel selected are highly skilled in the tasks for which they have been employed but, in time, it is discovered that they do not practice family-centered care. When this happens, it is important to address the problem as soon as possible. If the behavior cannot be changed, the executive must have the authority and ability to remove staff as well as hire them.

Leadership Teams

The nurse leader mentors, coaches, and works with the nursing management/leadership team. As with the nurse leader, team members must have a shared purpose and goals to which they are deeply committed (Senge, 1990). How the team communicates content, solves problems, and develops procedures for updating, linking, collaborating, and accountability are all crucial (Katzenbach & Smith, 1993; Robbins & Finley, 1995). The team members must also help and support each other as they make the necessary program changes.

Leadership Model

The nursing leadership team meets regularly to formulate plans, discuss issues related to program implementation, and address ongoing SRMC issues. These meetings also offer the opportunity to renew the team members' dedication to the SRMC program.

Recognizing that those who do the work are the most effective agents of change (Garcia, 1996), the clinical nurse manager and leadership team hold regular staff meetings. This permits the leadership team to provide information and encourage dialogue between leadership and staff. Staffing and scheduling issues and quality of care and human resource issues may also be discussed at these meetings.

The leadership team provides guidance, structure, process, and evaluation mechanisms for staff. They inform staff of committee actions and decisions. Good communication prevents rumors that can be highly damaging during the development of an SRMC program.

SRMC MARKETING AND COMMUNICATIONS

Marketing an SRMC program is one of the more interesting and rewarding challenges for a health care marketer. SRMC marketing is different from marketing of any other department or service within a hospital. This is not just because SRMC is a new service, but because it is a new kind of service.

A community survey will show little demand for SRMC. Five years ago, there was little demand for Internet access. Most people have never heard of single-room maternity care, but this does not mean that they will not want it, just as the population who did not know of the Internet is now appreciating and accessing it. SRMC addresses parents' desire for knowledge, support, and comfort during a major life transition. The large number of information sources that are supported by this interest—magazines, books, television shows, classes, and Internet sites—is an indication of the appetite that parents have for such information and support.

Unlike marketing a product or service that people already understand, SRMC marketing must first develop a community awareness of what an SRMC program is, what it brings to family beginnings, and how it differs from standard maternity care. To do this, marketers of SRMC must fully understand the components of care and the program by which it is provided.

How Not to Market SRMC

Instead of taking up the challenge of introducing new concepts, some SRMC marketing programs describe the beautiful rooms and high-quality medical and nursing care. However, beautiful rooms and high-quality care can be found in most maternity services today. Focusing on these features fails to differentiate SRMC from standard, high-quality maternity care and gives people no special reason to choose it.

Responsibility for SRMC Marketing

Effective marketing and communication are critical to the success of an SRMC program, because without community understanding it is difficult to accomplish either the social purposes of the maternity program or the marketing goals of the organization. A dedicated SRMC marketing function is necessary to ensure that a knowledgeable, sophisticated, and effective program is in place before, during, and after implementation of the new maternity service. As with all functions and processes within the SRMC program, marketing is the responsibility of the program developer until responsibility for the service is taken over by the SRMC administrator.

Strategic Marketing Focus

During strategic planning, it is especially important to have a strategic focus geared to meeting the family development goals of the SRMC program and to developing long-term family loyalty to the parent organization. Also, if SRMC services are to communicate the organization's commitment to family-centered care, the marketer should ensure that the organization's philosophy of care is written and communicated in support of the maternity service. The vision, values, and mission of the parent organization should be written to support the personalized, socially responsible, patient- and family-friendly care that

is provided in the SRMC unit. In reading the vision, values, and mission of the hospital, it should be easy to determine if they provide not just for a healthy bottom line but for the long-term definition necessary in the creation of a successful SRMC service.

Marketing Program Development

In securing a long-lasting relationship with families and their providers, the SRMC marketing includes relationship building, community support, and joint programming. Especially when resources are limited, it is often intangible external communications that most effectively promote the unique services of the facility and best convey the hospital's ability to serve the family's health continuum. If SRMC marketing efforts are built on a solid strategic foundation and supported by strong internal process and practice, external marketing initiatives will be the link necessary to drive and direct a successful SRMC program. SRMC internal and external marketing is directed toward provider and community goals.

Internal Marketing

Although the importance of marketing to the organization is often understated, in SRMC units it is essential. Everyone in the parent organization, not just those associated with the SRMC unit, must feel supportive of and connected to the maternity service's mission and activities.

Delivering the Promise

A prime marketing rule is: Don't promise what you can't deliver. The cost of any tangible marketing initiative will be completely lost and the SRMC unit reputation critically damaged if the hospital and unit do not actively support the SRMC care characterized in marketing communications. The SRMC marketer must understand the mindset and care philosophy of the providers who are responsible for care and must be continuously aware of the character and "feel" of the care that is provided.

Policies and procedures and observable care practice must be in harmony with the marketing program. Using the experienced input from the marketer, it is up to the SRMC administrator to ensure that personnel can not only provide SRMC care but also define it and exemplify it in their professional life. "Walking the talk" is crucial if personnel providing care and service to young families are to make a lasting impression. The mannerisms and attitudes reflected by the SRMC clinicians and facility appearance play major roles in the determination of patient satisfaction. Ultimately, it is that satisfaction that will determine whether the family returns to the hospital for the next phase of its healthcare development.

Clinical/Marketing Harmony

To enhance the relationship and understanding among providers, clinicians, and marketers of SRMC services, the marketer should actively participate in the unit operation, shadowing a variety of caregivers for a period of time and throughout various care stages. The result is an intimate understanding of both the philosophy of care and the actual operations on the unit.

Another way to develop understanding of the program is to follow families, with their permission, through the various stages in their care process. The marketer gathers information about what the family sees, hears, and feels in going through the various points of the care continuum. It is important for the marketer to attend some of the maternity educational sessions, because it is often enlightening to observe the sessions and then compare the content to what is actually promoted in the various marketing initiatives.

Participation in these activities gives the maternity service marketer a refined view of the product and the perspective necessary for specific and targeted communication. Most importantly, a collaborative relationship is developed between clinical staff and marketing, which fosters the necessary communication between the two entities. New developments in caregiving will not then be a surprise to the marketing department. Marketing initiatives will then be more easily understood, accepted, and implemented by the clinical staff.

Facility

The SRMC facility is not the prime product in the successful SRMC unit, but it is certainly a visual and instantly identifiable component (Figure 8-3). As described in Chapter 5, comfortable amenities and aesthetically soothing décor are part of creating a memorable and positive birth experience.

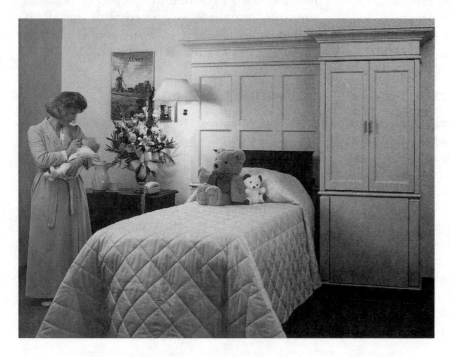

FIGURE 8–3. The SRMC facility is not the prime product in the successful SRMC unit, but it is certainly a visual and instantly identifiable component. (Photo courtesy of Legacy Good Samaritan Hospital, Portland, OR.)

The SRMC marketer, having intimate knowledge of the desires and needs of the service population, can provide significant input in the maintenance of the proper environment. Necessary signage, adequate privacy, and support areas for children and other family members are issues that must be addressed by the unit and that can impact marketing efforts.

Policies and procedures and observable care practice should be in harmony with the marketing program. Although the completion of registration paperwork and insurance discussions are a necessary part of any hospital stay, the family-supportive environment of the SRMC unit should offer private and practical areas for the patient's completion of such procedures. Clinician involvement in any marketing initiative required during the birthing and family development process (baby photos, distribution of hospital incentives, baby web site registrations) should be thoughtfully and strategically planned, combining as many steps as possible and minimizing time away from patient care.

Incentive

Although knowing that providing SRMC is the "right thing to do" is sufficient motivation for healthcare professionals, recognition of the superior care provided by SRMC staff is important. Responsibilities and privileges depend on attainment of skills, and these are appropriately recognized. For example, nursing staff who have demonstrated a required level of core and specialty skills are identified. Physicians who have gained privileges to practice on the SRMC service are identified in the unit's promotional material and receive referrals from the unit's referral line. Consumer feedback can also be an important reinforcer of family-centered maternity practices.

External Communications Plan

External marketing goals include:

- To create community awareness of what an SRMC program is, what it brings to family beginnings, and how it differs from standard maternity care

- To develop community support for the SRMC program among individuals and community organizations
- To make SRMC goals personally relevant to prospective clients, and to develop an expectation that SRMC should be available to them
- To motivate parents-to-be to seek out SRMC and to provide easy access to SRMC
- To generate long-term loyalty to the service and to the parent hospital

Advertising

Advertising, although not the only necessary type of external communication, is important to develop community awareness of the new SRMC program. Even the most conservative marketing plan should include a variety of products. Brochures, flyers, direct mail pieces, radio, TV, and print advertisements should all be considered. The most critical thing to remember about SRMC advertisements is that they should be targeted to family development and creatively designed to complement the unique SRMC program. All efforts and products should have a common theme, being part of an overall strategic campaign. Through a series of external communications and media, the marketer should plan focused outreach to prospective families, providers, and the community. Efforts should center on long-term relationship building, education, and communication.

Community Understanding of SRMC

Developing community awareness is not the same as developing community understanding. SRMC is not an easy concept to explain on a billboard. Advertising and billboards create little more than awareness and curiosity. Curiosity will not abide a vacuum. If you do not define what SRMC is when it is first introduced, the community or your competitors will define it for you. Attention-getting advertising must be closely connected with and supported by information that creates an understanding of what SRMC is (Figures 8-4 to 8-6).

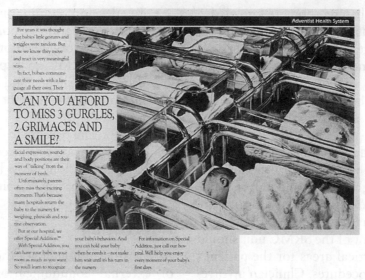

FIGURE 8–4. A print ad focusing on the benefits of mother-baby nursing.

In determining a long-term market strategy, the marketer begins with the determination of where the community is in terms of knowledge and expectations. Information gathered during the strategic planning process forms a baseline toward which marketing efforts are attuned and from which progress toward developing community understanding can be measured. Promotional efforts are planned to reach defined objectives over a period of years, based on community receptivity and the overall strategy plans of the hospital and the SRMC unit.

The message of SRMC is planned to resonate with the community's desire for knowledge, support, and care during the childbearing year. Marketing must differentiate SRMC from conventional maternity services, explaining its focus on parental empowerment and family development.

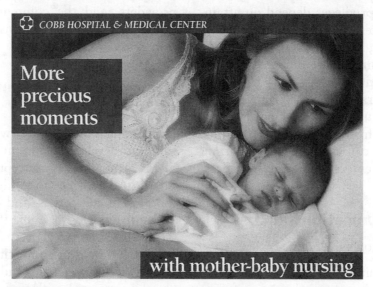

FIGURE 8–5. A brochure describing more precious moments with mother–baby nursing. (Photo courtesy of Wellstar Cobb Medical Center, Austell, GA.)

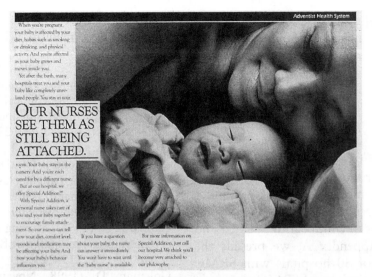

FIGURE 8–6. A print ad with primary focus on the family-centered care model of mother-baby nursing.

This requires sensitivity and sophistication to communicate a complex message and to avoid the social and political landmines that occur in any field of social change. In using public relations efforts as a prime component in external marketing, the marketer should take the time to ensure that those people responsible for communicating can easily and with passion define the uniqueness of SRMC.

Community Education

There are many effective ways to educate the community about SRMC, including providing speakers to civic organizations, community groups, schools, and colleges. Childbirth education classes are often the expecting family's first entry to the SRMC process. The marketer should work closely with the education director to ensure that a message consistent with the philosophy of care, the external communications, and the actual care process is communicated. The very first education experience for the prospective patient should demonstrate that SRMC is not a typical program. Participants should walk away believing they have just experienced the initial step in their family development process.

SRMC prenatal education is different from conventional childbirth preparation in its focus on parent participation, education, and empowerment, and on content addressing physiologic labor and birth and family development. Although childbirth education is a component of care, not a marketing device, it can be highly effective in developing community awareness of, and demand for, SRMC.

PROCESS EVALUATION

Important yet often forgotten in the marketing process is evaluation of the effectiveness of the marketing procedures used. Patient satisfaction surveys are a good method of determining the overall success of the care process. Interviewing parents selected at random after they have settled into their new family roles is better, because reactions are less influenced by the excitement of the birth. The survey tool includes all areas of the care process—from entry into the system, registration, education, provider and clinician care review, security, facility, and amenities. Most importantly, the outcomes are consistently analyzed to determine the direction of future marketing efforts. An additional method of evaluation is the tracking of referrals to the hospital. It is the hope of all SRMC administrators that patients will be guided to the facility by positive word of mouth. Although that may be the case in many instances, it is very helpful to determine the source of patient referral. Consistently tracking patient patterns will help the administrator and marketer determine where best to invest crucial marketing resources.

SUMMARY

SRMC holds the promise of providing quality maternity care in a more cost-effective manner than traditional maternity care models, while better meeting the needs of childbearing women and their families. In Appendix A, we present the results of a survey of 30 hospitals with SRMC programs. Brief descriptions of SRMC programs selected from those who participated in the survey follow in Appendix B. It is clear that realizing the promise, however, requires crafting an organizational structure that takes into account the unique demands of SRMC programs. It also means rethinking conventional operational methods and staffing patterns so as to make intelligent and appropriate use of all resources and categories of staff. Interrelationships are revamped so that authority derives from experience, ability, and example. Nonetheless, the achievement is well worth the effort: an organization where all staff members can participate to the fullest extent of their training and skill in serving women, infants, and their families.

REFERENCES

American Academy of Pediatrics & American College of Obstetricians and Gynecologists. (1997). *Guidelines for perinatal care* (4th ed.). Elk Grove, IL: American Academy of Pediatrics.

Association of Women's Health, Obstetric and Neonatal Nurses. (1997). Issue: The role of unlicensed assistive personnel in the nursing care for women and newborns. Position paper.

Barter, M., McLaughlin, F. E., & Thomas, S. A. (1994). Use of unlicensed assistive personnel by hospitals. *Nursing Economic$, 12*(2), 82–87.

Blancett, S. S., & Flarey, D. L. (1995). *Reengineering nursing and health care: The handbook for organizational transformation.* Gaithersburg, MD: Aspen.

Blegen, M. A., Goode, C. J., & Reed, L. (1998). Nurse staffing and patient outcomes. *Nursing Research, 47*(1), 43–50.

Bond, G. E., & Fiedler, F. E. (1999). A comparison of leadership vs. renovation in changing staff values. *Nursing Economic$, 17*(1), 37–43.

Duclos-Miller, P. A. (1996). Workload measurement tracking system. *Nursing Management, 27*(9), 39–41.

Fitzgerald, K. (1998). Clinical benchmarking: Implications for perinatal nursing. *Journal of Perinatal Neonatal Nursing, 12*(1), 23–30.

Freitas, C. A., Helmer, F. T., & Cousins, N. (1987, September/October). The development and management uses of a patient classification system for a high-risk perinatal center. *Journal Of Obstetric Gynecologic and Neonatal Nursing, 17*, 330–338.

Garcia, E. A. (1996). Moving change through the system: A model for staff involvement. *Maternity Child Nursing, 21*, 219–221.

Goleman, D. (1998, November/December). What makes a leader? *Harvard Business Review,* 93–102

Hines, P. A. P., Smeltzer, C. H., & Galletti, M. (1994). Work restructuring: The process of redefining roles of patient caregivers. *Nursing Economic$, 12*(6), 346–350.

Irvine, D., Sidani, S., & Hall, L. M. (1998). Linking outcomes to nurses' roles in health care. *Nursing Economic$, 16*(2), 58–64, 87.

Jones, D., Famularo, B. E., Desta, T. F., Fulgencio, A. A., & Rotondo, L. (1992). A labor and delivery service unit model for a multihospital health maintenance organization. *Nursing Economic$, 10*(2), 127–134.

Katzenbach, J. R., & Smith, D. K. (1993). *The wisdom of teams: Creating the high-performance organization.* New York: HarperBusiness.

Kovner, C., & Gergen, P. J. (1998). Nurse staffing levels and adverse events following surgery in US hospitals. *Image: Journal of Nursing Scholarship, 30*(4), 315–321.

Krapohl, G. L., & Larson, E. (1996). The impact of unlicensed assistive personnel on nursing care delivery. *Nursing Economic$, 14*(2), 99–110.

Lengacher, C. A., Kent, K., Mabe, P. R., Heinemann, D., Van Cott, M. L., & Bowling, C. D. (1994). Effects of the partners in care practice model on nursing outcomes. *Nursing Economic$, 12*(6), 300–308.

Lengacher, C. A., Mabe, P. R., Bowling, C. D., Heinemann, D., Kent, K., & Van Cott, M. L. (1993). Redesigning nursing practice: The partners in patient care model. *Journal of Nursing Administration, 23*(12), 31–37.

Loveridge, C. E., & Cummings, S. H. (1996). *Nursing management in the new paradigm.* Gaithersburg, MD: Aspen.

O'Toole, J. (1995). *Leading change: Overcoming the ideology of comfort and the tyranny of custom.* San Francisco: Jossey-Bass.

Phillips, C. R. (1988). Productivity and maternity nursing. *Nursing Management, 19*(10), 54–59.

Pischke-Winn, K., & Minnick, A. (1996). Project management: Lessons learned from introducing a multitask environmental worker program. *Journal of Nursing Administration, 26*(6), 31–38.

Robbins, H., & Finley, M. (1995). *Why teams don't work: What went wrong and how to make it right.* Princeton, NJ: Peterson's/Pacesetter Books.

Schmid, M., & Gerlach, C. (1986). LDRP: Staffing a single care maternity system. *Nursing Management, 17*(8), 36–40.

Schwamb, J. (1989). A maternity patient classification system. *Nursing Management, 20*(11), 66, 70–71.

Senge, P. M. (1990). *The fifth discipline: The art and practice of the learning organization.* New York: Currency Doubleday.

Stenske, J., & Ferguson, R. (1996) Analysis of labor and delivery workload. *Nursing Management, 27*(6), 30–32.

In Conclusion

Single-room maternity care is the logical program for the 21st century. SRMC has a wellness and prevention orientation, utilizes collaborative multidisciplinary teams of providers, and the facility design promotes efficient, cost-effective, noninterventive maternity practices. The value-added component of SRMC is that when properly designed and implemented, SRMC offers the promise of better family beginnings.

Early indications are that comprehensive SRMC programs are highly valued. If enough consumers learn about and want comprehensive family-oriented maternity care, health plans will need to offer it in order to be competitive. However, maternity care cannot usually survive as a stand-alone service, and neither is it in the community's best interest that it do so. The childbearing year is only the beginning of a series of vital transitions to be made during development of the family, and providers of maternity care are well positioned to expand family care through the childbearing and childcare years in collaboration with other providers.

The maternity industry's next mission could be to facilitate the development of stronger, more knowledgeable, and competent families through the provision of socially responsible care during the childbearing year. Maternity care professional organizations have long called for the provision of family-centered care. Most maternity care professionals believe in family-centered maternity care. If we believe that birth is foremost the beginning of a family, it follows that we are in the business of family beginnings. In SRMC, we have a mission, a method, and a means to serve this business. All that the maternity care system needs is the motivation to take the next step.

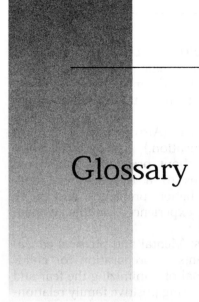

Glossary

acquaintance: Process of getting to know the newborn; includes bonding and initial attachment.

analgesia: Pain relief without loss of consciousness.

anesthesia: A loss of sensation, especially to pain, with or without loss of consciousness.

attachment: A feeling of affection or loyalty that binds one person to another, which occurs at critical periods, such as birth or adoption. It is unique, specific, and enduring, and follows bonding.

birth plan: A plan or a list of options a pregnant woman and her partner design regarding the type of childbirth experience she would like to have (minimal medical intervention, presence of family members, monitoring, position in labor, breastfeeding, pain relief, and so forth).

birthing room: A private space, within a hospital, designed for only low-risk childbearing families to labor and birth.

bonding: The initial stage in a relationship characterized by a strong attraction and a desire to interact.

certified nurse-midwife (CNM): A registered nurse with special postgraduate preparation in gynecology and obstetrics, qualified to independently manage the care of essentially normal women and newborns before, during, and after birth and/or gynecologically.

clinical nurse specialist (CNS): A registered nurse who has become expert at the graduate level in a defined area of knowledge and practice in nursing.

conventional maternity care: An obstetric model that utilizes the multitransfer system of either delivery rooms or LDRs.

culture: The sum of a group of people's values, beliefs, and practices that are transmitted from one generation to the next.

developmental task: A necessary step in growth and maturation that one must complete before additional growth and maturation are possible.

doula: A trained, experienced woman who supports the laboring woman one-to-one, providing reassurance, encouragement, stroking her, holding her hand, walking with her, suggesting position changes, instructing her, and instructing and reassuring her partner.

evidence-based practice (EBP): An approach to healthcare in which health professionals use the best evidence possible, that is, the most appropriate information available, to make clinical decisions for individual patients. In practical terms, that means basing patient care on more than tradition, that is, "we've always done it that way."

family: In FCMC, the family includes those persons the childbearing woman identifies as providing familial support, whether or not they are biologically related.

FCMC (family-centered maternity care): A consumer-focused approach to maternity care that places emphasis on the childbearing woman within the context of her family.

LDR room (labor, delivery, recovery): A component of a multitransfer system that combines labor, delivery, and recovery functions in one room. The family is then moved to postpartum.

LDRP room (labor, delivery, recovery, postpartum): A component of an SRMC system in which multiskilled nurses provide care to the women without moving them.

midwife: A person other than a physician who is trained to assist women in childbirth. The training may be either formal or informal. Two kinds of midwives practice in the United States: certified nurse-midwives and lay midwives (also called independent midwives).

monitrice: A person trained in psychoprophylactic methods and who attends women during labor.

mother–baby nursing: A model of maternity nursing in which one multiskilled nurse provides care for the mother and baby together.

nurse anesthetist: A registered nurse who has advanced education and certification in administering anesthetics. Also known as certified registered nurse anesthetist (CRNA).

nurse practice acts: Laws that determine the scope of nursing practice in each state.

nurse practitioner (NP): A registered nurse with advanced preparation that allows him or her to provide primary care for specific groups of patients. All nurse practitioners collaborate with physicians for treatments and medications within their scope of practice.

obstetrics: That branch of medicine defined as the art and science of caring for the childbearing woman and her unborn baby.

parent institution: The source and controlling organization, or the organization from which a stand-alone program or facility has been produced.

perinatal: The time period from the 20th week of pregnancy to 4 weeks after childbirth.

physician champion: A physician who fights for and supports the organization's clinical program design, mission, and vision.

physiologic childbirth: A clinical approach to childbirth management that utilizes the mother's physical and emotional capabilities and her support systems to the fullest extent possible.

prepared childbirth: (Also natural childbirth or childbirth education.) A program of prenatal education about pregnancy, labor, and birth as a means to a less anxious, more knowledgeable, better prepared, and more satisfying birth experience for the woman and her partner.

psychoprophylaxis: Mental and physical education of the parents in preparation for childbirth, with the goal of minimizing the fear and pain and of promoting positive family relationships.

role transition: Changing from one pattern of behavior and one image of self to another.

rooming-in: A maternity care model in which the baby may remain in the mother's postpartum room. Postpartum nurses care for the mother, and nursery nurses provide infant care.

SRMC (single-room maternity care): A care program and facility plan designed to facilitate the provision of family-centered maternity care in a nontransfer setting.

SRMC cluster: An SRMC unit's clinical care model. It is comprised of LDRP rooms surrounding a central service nursing core.

standard of care: Level of care that can be expected of a professional.

umbilical connection to hospital services: A formal agreement that provides support and services between a freestanding SRMC facility and program and the parent organization. The object is to provide seamless services so the two organizations appear as one.

VBAC: Vaginal birth after a cesarean.

women's center: A hospital-based service for women's ambulatory care and diagnostic services. May be on- or off-campus.

women's specialty "mini-hospital": An independent hospital that provides specialty care for women. In addition to ambulatory care and diagnostics, the specialty women's hospital may provide maternity, surgical, and other services. It may be allied with other hospitals as part of a larger healthcare organization.

SRMC Programs[*]

In January 1999, Phillips+Fenwick mailed a questionnaire to 50 maternity units that practice Single-Room Maternity Care (SRMC) in various regions of the nation. Although there are hundreds of SRMC units nationally, the 50 selected for inclusion in our mailing practice in a manner that we perceived to be consistent with the SRMC philosophy that has been articulated throughout this book. We sought to determine whether these units validate our beliefs about the benefits of SRMC practice. We mailed surveys to 50 obstetrical units, and 30 completed surveys were returned to us (response rate = 60%). Of those 30 respondents, 22 answered the survey fully, and 8 responded to some questions and not to others. In the following commentary, the number responding to each question will be noted along with each finding.

The limited findings presented in this summary are intended as a descriptive exercise of the features that characterize a small sampling of good SRMC programs nationally. The SRMC programs included in the analysis are typical of program diversity nationally. Some have been operational for several years, others are new. Some have upgraded from the multitransfer system,

others initiated their entry into obstetrics with an SRMC unit. Respondents are part of large and small hospitals, ranging in size from 28 to 608 beds. Seventy-two percent are affiliated with systems. The commonalties among them are that they all practice SRMC, and all their nursing staffs function in either mother–baby nursing or all three maternity care specialty areas.

DEMOGRAPHIC FACTORS

Several demographic/descriptive variables were included in the questionnaire for categorization and descriptive purposes. These included a variety of questions regarding level of care, size of hospital, region of the country in which the hospital is located, and so on.

Responses by Region

The SRMC model of care was first implemented in the Midwest in the late 1970s as a means of cutting costs and increasing market share in an emerging managed care environment. Shortly after, hospitals in the South also developed

---

[*]Study by Elizabeth Hamilton, PhD.

SRMC units. Although managed care had not extended as prominently to the southern region of the country, SRMC was viewed as a means of increasing consumer satisfaction with hospital-based maternity programs and as a way to differentiate one program from another when marketing to consumers. Other regions of the country embraced the SRMC philosophy of care more gradually, and it eventually spread to every region of the nation.

Given the historic evolution of SRMC units, it is not surprising to find that even though the Phillips+Fenwick survey was sent to all regions of the nation, the Midwest and South were most highly represented in responses. Figure A-1 graphically indicates the percentage of responses from each region. Regional designations are based on definitions used by the U.S. Census Bureau.

Number of Deliveries in 1998

As SRMC evolved, so too did myths about the appropriateness of the care model. In particular, it was frequently stated that SRMC was appropriate only for small, low-risk environments. That particular myth is dashed by about 20% of the hospitals that responded to this survey, for they are hospitals operating successful obstetrical units in Level III and, in some cases Level IV, perinatal

environments and delivering in excess of 3000 babies per year. The distribution of 1998 deliveries is shown in Figure A-2 for sample hospitals.

PROGRAM

In addition to the units' demographic characteristics, we were interested in perceptions regarding clinical safety and family and staff satisfaction since changing care models. These questions were derived from other myths about SRMC: that SRMC was not as clinically safe as the multi-transfer model of care, that families were less satisfied in an SRMC environment, and that staff satisfaction declined in an SRMC unit.

Clinical Safety

Respondents were asked to state how clinical safety compared with that noted in the previous care model. Hospitals with new start-up OB units had no basis for comparison and did not respond to this question. In some cases, the individual responding to the question had not been a staff member at the time of the change and could not answer the question. Twenty-one hospitals did respond, as shown in Figure A-3. Almost half

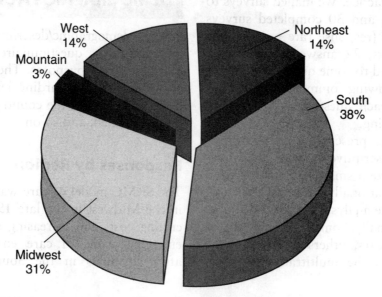

FIGURE A-1. Percentage of responses from each region of the U.S.

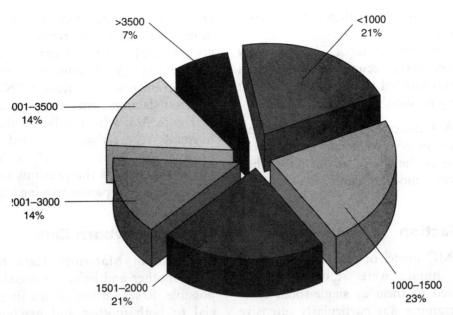

FIGURE A–2. 1998 births at responding hospitals. (n = 29)

found safety to be at least equivalent to that under the multitransfer system, and the remaining 52% perceived safety to be either "better" or "much better" than it had been under the previous system of care.

Response to Family Needs

A family-centered approach to care is a key element of the SRMC model of care. The birth of a child is not something that happens to a woman, it happens to a family. Therefore, in-

cluding family members chosen by the laboring woman enhances the process for all of them. The presence of family members has been shown to augment the birthing experience for all participants, caregivers as well as family members.

- Caregivers have an opportunity to bond with the family and to observe family members interacting with one another and the newborn.
- Family members can be educated about newborn care and can bond with the newborn in

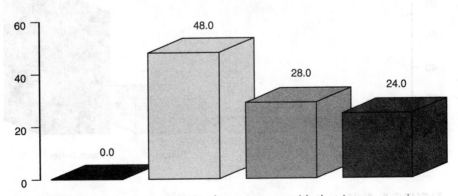

FIGURE A–3. How does clinical safety compare with that in your previous care model? (n = 21)

the mother's room rather than in the less private nursery setting.

- The woman, both in labor and as a new mother, feels more secure with loved ones who she has selected to be present either at the delivery or shortly thereafter.

As Figure A-4 indicates, survey respondents were unanimous in perceiving that family needs were better met in the SRMC environment than under the previous model of care.

Staff Satisfaction

When the SRMC model of care was first suggested, some nurses were resistant to the changes required of them as single-room caregivers. Cross-training was particularly offensive to many who feared they would be less effective in both their former area of specialty and the new area to which they were being educated. Other nurses objected to caring for a type of patient whom they had not selected as a specialty level when they first became maternity nursing professionals. Those who cared for postpartum mothers were reluctant to care for newborns and vice versa. Among the 24 hospitals that responded to the staff satisfaction question, 24% experienced staff turnover as a result of the change in care models. Only one hospital reported that staff turnover is still a problem. Close to 30% reported that most nurses are

cross-trained to postpartum nursery with a separate L&D staff. The remaining 70% are fully cross-trained to three areas (L&D, postpartum, and nursery). Many units also care for high-risk antepartum patients and/or GYN surgical cases. Staff satisfaction with current positions is shown in Figure A-5, which indicates that 92% of the hospitals report that staff satisfaction is either "better" or "much better" under the SRMC model than under the previous care model that featured three separate nursing staffs.

Type of Newborn Care

Single-Room Maternity Care functions best when mother and baby are together as much as possible. Research has shown that this is beneficial to both mother and newborn physiologically, but it is important educationally as well. Having the baby present in her room gives the new mother opportunities to learn about her newborn in a safe environment in which she can ask questions. She is also better able to learn the baby's sleep patterns and idiosyncrasies prior to being discharged. Although ideally the infant is with its mother most of the time, the new mother does have an option to send the baby to a respite area for short periods of time if she so desires.

The SRMC model features mother–baby nursing care. In this type of care, one nurse cares for both mother and baby. For this reason, it is

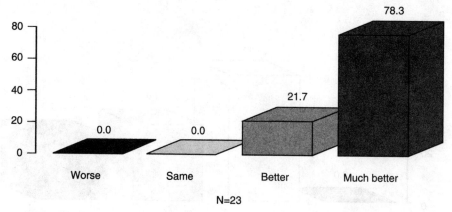

FIGURE A–4. How does current response to family needs compare with that in your previous care model?

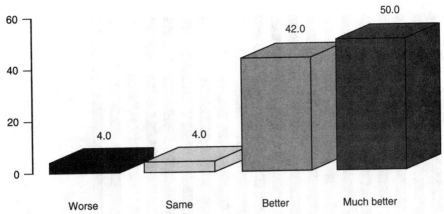

FIGURE A–5. How does staff satisfaction compare with that in your previous care model? (n = 24)

sometimes termed "coupled care." In contrast, "rooming in" requires the mother and family members to care for the newborn while he or she is in the room; a nursery nurse cares for the infant in the nursery. As shown in Figure A-6, none of the 29 hospitals that responded to the newborn care question currently have rooming-in as a feature of their program, and only a small percentage feature a conventional newborn nursery with separate nursery staff. About 96% practice mother–baby nursing, 72% of units operate with mother–baby nursing and a respite area,

and about 24% practice mother–baby nursing and maintain a separate newborn nursery, frequently because state regulations require them to do so.

Percentage of Time Baby Is With Mother

Responses varied among the 22 hospitals that answered questions regarding the time that the baby is in the mother's room following delivery. During daytime hours, most babies are in the rooms. Figure A-7 indicates the distribution of

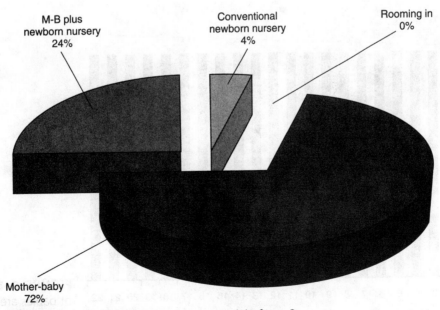

FIGURE A–6. What is the newborn model of care?

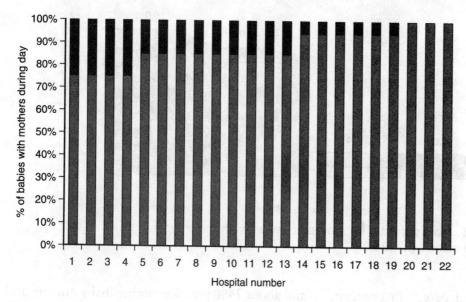

FIGURE A–7. Percent of babies who are with their mothers during the day, by hospital.

babies with mothers in each hospital during day-time hours. The graphic indicates that:

- At four hospitals, a minimum of 75% of babies are with mothers during the day.
- At nine hospitals, a minimum of 85% of babies are with mothers during the day.
- At six hospitals, a minimum of 95% of babies are with mothers during the day.
- At three hospitals, 100% of babies are with mothers during the daytime hours.

Figure A-8 indicates that of the 22 hospitals responding to this question, there is a good deal of variation in the percentage of babies spending nighttime hours in mothers' rooms.

- Two hospitals reported less than 35% of infants with mothers at night.
- Two hospitals reported about 40% of infants with mothers at night.
- Four hospitals reported 55% of infants with mothers at night.

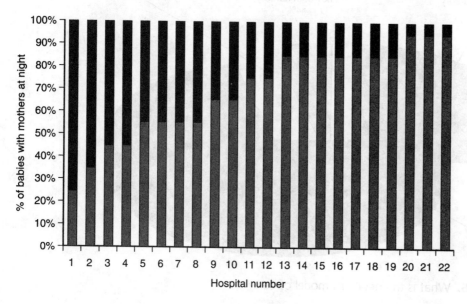

FIGURE A–8. What percent of babies are with their mothers at night?

- Two hospitals reported 65% of infants with mothers at night.
- Two hospitals reported 75% of infants with mothers at night.
- Seven hospitals reported 85% of infants with mothers at night.
- Three hospitals reported 95% of infants with mothers at night.

Education

Ideally, the principles of family-centered care are a well-integrated part of an SRMC program. Family-centered care principles point to each woman's individuality and comment upon each woman's differing educational needs, both in preparing for labor and delivery and following birth. To assess this dimension in the care continuum, we presented a checklist to respondents and asked them to select those services that were offered as part of their obstetrical program.

Table A-1 indicates that 100% of the 30 programs offer childbirth education, 97% offer lactation education, and close to 80% have some type of home care program available for the post-discharge care of new mothers and their normal newborns. Some also have home health care options for NICU babies following discharge. Slightly more than half offer doula services.

TABLE A–1 ■ OPPORTUNITIES FOR EDUCATION (N = 30)

Educational Opportunity	N	Percent
Childbirth education	30	100.0
Lactation education	28	96.6
Home health care—postpartum	23	79.3
Home health care—newborn	23	79.3
Home health care—antenatal	18	62.1
Early discharge program	17	58.6
Doula	15	51.7
Home health care—NICU	14	48.3

MARKETING

The tendency of some hospitals to view SRMC as a marketing tool through which they could differentiate their maternity product from that of competitors was mentioned earlier in this report. In fact, the observation was validated through respondent answers to a question regarding their motivation for changing to an SRMC care model. Sixty-four percent stated that the program was changed to SRMC to influence market share. The second most frequently cited reason for switching was to "be first to have SRMC" (22%).

In the early days of SRMC, the marketing advantage was perceived to be large LDRP rooms and a warm, homey décor. As the model was more fully integrated nationally, marketers discovered that it was not only the rooms that gave SRMC its differentiating appeal. The way that people were treated in an SRMC environment also had an impact. This is evidenced by the fact that consumer satisfaction increased dramatically when families experienced SRMC programs.

Consumer Satisfaction

For 96% of respondents, customer satisfaction is measured through a formal process involving a hospital satisfaction questionnaire or some type of pre-post test analysis. Only 4% rely upon personal perception to determine client satisfaction.

According to these formalized measurement tools, customer satisfaction is better with the current SRMC program than it was with the former program. Of the 96% reporting improved customer happiness with services, 77% reported "much better" satisfaction, and 19% said customer satisfaction was "somewhat better." Based on that response, 97% confidently called their OB program "successful." Moreover, 75% of respondents stated that obstetrics was not considered a loss leader at their hospitals (N = 21).

Eighty-nine percent of the units responding (N = 27) said that their OB program has a distinct identity, 77% have a positioning strategy for the program, and 85% have a formal marketing plan.

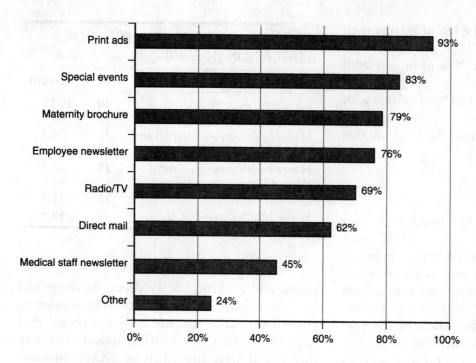

FIGURE A–9. Percent employing each type of marketing medium. (n = 30) (*Note:* Multiple-response question; percentages do not total 100%.)

Marketing Media Preferences

Many marketing media are used to convey the SRMC message. Figure A-9 indicates the media preferences of the 29 hospitals that responded to this part of the survey.

SUMMARY

This small-sample, self-report survey has indicated the following among most hospitals that have changed to SRMC programs:

- Consumer satisfaction, as measured by formal surveys, is higher.
- Responsiveness to the needs of families is improved.
- Clinical safety is the same or better than it was previously.
- Staff satisfaction has increased.
- A higher percentage of mothers and babies are remaining together following delivery.
- Education is stressed both prior to labor and delivery and following discharge from the hospital.

Surveyed Hospitals

There are hundreds of hospitals providing SRMC throughout the United States. Following are key program points from some of the hospitals included in the Phillips+Fenwick survey in Appendix A. Represented here are examples of successful SRMC programs.

In general, these hospital SRMC programs share the commonalities of consumer satisfaction, staff satisfaction, family-centered philosophies and programming, multiskilled nursing staff, recognition for excellence in patient care, improvements in payer mix and market share, collaborative practice, comprehensive education programs for new parents and families, and the message that redesigning maternity care is never finished. Each SRMC program continually strives for excellence.

Even relatively simple developments within industries take time to establish themselves, work out the kinks, and gain sufficient consumer awareness and trust to modify ingrained cultures and behaviors. There are no perfect SRMC programs. However, there is a lot to be learned from these pioneers.

HOSPITALS WITH LESS THAN 1,000 BPY

- Dartmouth-Hitchcock Medical Center
- Family Maternity Center, Saint Alphonsus Regional Medical Center
- Illini Hospital
- Seacoast Birth Center, Anna Jaques Hospital
- Sutter Maternity and Surgery Center
- Williamsburg Community Hospital

Dartmouth-Hitchcock Medical Center
One Medical Center Drive
Lebanon, NH 03756-0001

410-bed hospital
Level III SRMC Maternity Service
Level IV Newborn Service
17 LDRPs

- Listed in *Self* magazine's "America's 10 Best Hospitals When You Are Having a Baby" (December 1996).

- "Our philosophy is that birth and pregnancy are life events, not medical events. We believe that medicine can help. We're here to facilitate, as consultants. But we're not here to tell you what your social and cultural needs are surrounding birth."
- A successful marriage between progressive attitudes and cutting-edge technology has long kept Dartmouth-Hitchcock among the handful of the country's best. An example: Although it serves as a regional high-risk center and maintains a respected intensive care nursery, Hitchcock does not isolate its high-risk patients. Instead, it has managed to blend the high-tech care right into the rest of the birthing pavilion, helping high-risk patients feel as if they are part of the normal birthing community.
- OB/GYNs and nurse-midwives are so well integrated that when a complication occurs with a midwife-attended birth, the physician does not simply take over the case; the doctor and the midwife co-manage.

Family Maternity Center
Saint Alphonsus Regional Medical Center
1055 N. Curtis Road
Boise, ID 83706

281-bed hospital
Level II SRMC Maternity Service
Level II Newborn Service
12 LDRPs

- This is a new maternity service that started in 1997.

Philosophy Statement

Consistent with the values of Sisters of the Holy Cross and in support of the strategic vision of Saint Alphonsus, we share with and support families in the birth of new life through a partnership of technology and personal care.

You and your family will:

- Be our highest priority
- Receive our respect and compassion
- Receive excellent, competent care

Our professional team will:

- Value sharing in your birth experience
- Work for the benefit of you and your family
- Include you and your family in the planning and delivery of care

Mission Statement

Family-centered maternity care is consistent with the values of the Holy Cross and in support of the strategic vision of Saint Alphonsus Regional Medical Center; we share with and support families in the birth of new life through a partnership of technology and personal care.

Vision Statement

Guided by the mission and core values of Sisters of the Holy Cross, the Family Maternity Center at Saint Alphonsus Regional Medical Center is the preferred choice of the community we serve.

Family Support Program—Scope and Purpose

The purpose of the family support nurse is to plan, coordinate, and implement activities and programs that facilitate wellness and ensure appropriateness of care for the families that access our services, including:

- Care planning
- Care conference
- Bereavement counseling
- QI/QA
- Community relations

Family Support Program Assumptions

- The client will identify their own family structure.
- Functional families contribute to the wellness of each member.
- Birth of a new member precipitates a developmental crisis.
- Positive resolution of the crisis strengthens the family unit.

- It is congruent with the mission of SARMC to strengthen families.
- A percentage of the Family Maternity Center population will require intervention pre- and post-inpatient stay.
- Primary prevention of suboptimal outcomes will pay for the family support program.

Family Support Program Components

- Preadmission assessments
- Physical
- Psychological
- Psychosocial
- Discharge
- Care and collaboration
- Patient and family education
- Anticipatory
- Tertiary

Illini Hospital
801 Hospital Road
Silvis, IL 61282

The Family Room
133-bed hospital
Level II SRMC Maternity Service
Level II Newborn Service
10 LDRPs

- Converted conventional multitransfer OB service to SRMC in 1986.
- 100% multiskilled nursing staff.

Seacoast Birth Center
Anna Jaques Hospital
25 Highland Avenue
Newburyport, MA 01950

156-bed hospital
Level II SRMC Maternity Service
Level IB Newborn Service (Continuing Care Facility per Massachusetts designation)
10 LDRPs

- High degree of patient satisfaction.
- Hospital is best known for maternity and newborn care.

- A physician champion motivated the hospital change to SRMC.

Mission Statement/Philosophy

- The Seacoast Birth Center is an integral component of the Anna Jaques Hospital.
- The center plays an important role in promoting health and is a vital community resource for women's health issues and family living. The quality and appropriateness of services provided to the center's clientele are monitored in an ongoing and systematic manner in order to promote high-quality patient care; to act on opportunities to improve the level and delivery of care; and to resolve identified problems or issues.
- Family-centered care has been the foundation of the Seacoast Birth Center. This comprehensive and personalized care concept is further enhanced by the collaboration and the teamwork among the members of the perinatal team.
- The single-room maternity care concept provides the patient and her family the privacy they seek and allows the staff to provide a continuum of care that is less fragmented and cost-effective.
- The various programs designed and implemented by the staff reflect the wide range of services for the community from direct patient care to different forms of patient education and support.
- The center's comprehensive program on lactation under the aegis of the Seacoast Birth Center Lactation Connection exemplifies many successes consistent with the quality of service and competence of its staff.

Program

- At the Seacoast Birth Center, single-room maternity care allows for a family-centered birth experience that truly caters to the personal needs of each mother, baby, and family.
- Labor, delivery, recovery, and postpartum (LDRP) care all take place in a single, private

room. State-of-the-art obstetric medical equipment is ready for use but concealed behind closed doors. A luxurious and relaxing ambiance promotes a sense of well-being for all.

- Fathers or significant others are encouraged to participate in the entire birth experience. A comfortable reclining lounger in every room provides for overnight stays.
- Each room has a refrigerator and stereo system as well as its own private bathroom complete with shower. A Jacuzzi room is also available to soothe and relax mothers in labor.
- The Seacoast Birth Center also features state-of-the-art medical technology with facilities for cesarean deliveries. They take pride in being one of the very few hospitals in New England with a low cesarean birth rate. (Primary = 10%; repeat cesarean = 6%.)
- There are several options in pain management, from relaxation techniques to epidural anesthesia with an anesthesiologist in-house 24 hours a day.
- The Seacoast Birth Center nurses are trained and skilled in all areas of maternity and newborn care and serve as teachers and as sources of emotional support for the mother and her family. The same nurse each shift is assigned to both mother and baby—not only to provide expert clinical care, but also to better coordinate nursing care.

Sutter Maternity and Surgery Center
2900 Chanticleer Avenue
Santa Cruz, CA 95065

Freestanding 30-bed specialty hospital
Level I SRMC Maternity Service
Level I Newborn Service
12 LDRPs

- New freestanding hospital, opened in 1996.
- Consumers say: "Feels more like a five-star hotel with the safety net of a hospital."
- Parkside patient satisfaction surveys are consistently the highest in the country.
- 100% of babies are with their mothers day and night.
- 100% multiskilled nursing staff.

Williamsburg Community Hospital
301 Monticello Avenue
Williamsburg, VA 23187

139-bed hospital
Level I SRMC Maternity Service
Level I Newborn Service
11 LDRPs

- Women are encouraged to ambulate in early labor, use showers for hydrotherapy, assume multiple positions during labor, and use a birthing ball during labor.

HOSPITALS WITH 1,000 TO 1,500 BPY

- Carroll County General Hospital, Inc.
- The Family Place, Concord Hospital
- The Good Samaritan Hospital, Lebanon, PA
- Harbor Hospital Center
- Mercy Health Partners, Fairfield Hospital
- Via Christi Regional Medical Center, St. Joseph Campus

Carroll County General Hospital, Inc.
200 Memorial Avenue
Westminster, MD 21157

Family Birth Place
168-bed hospital
Level II SRMC Maternity Service
Level II Newborn Service
10 LDRPs

- Ranked in the top 10% of a nationwide survey ranking 400 hospitals.
- Known for "family-centered" approach.
- Converted a traditional multitransfer OB service to SRMC in 1996.
- 95% of babies are with their mothers day and night.

The Family Place
Concord Hospital
250 Pleasant Street
Concord, NH 03301

180-bed hospital
Level II SRMC Maternity Service
Level II Newborn Service
18 LDRPs

- Center of excellence for patient-focused comprehensive LDRP care in the Northeast.
- 100% multiskilled staff.

Philosophy

- We believe that birth is a normal, healthy life event.
- We believe that the birth process may occasionally require medical assistance in ensuring a healthy outcome.
- We believe that women have a significant influence in healthcare decision making and need to be informed in order to make these decisions.
- We believe that women's healthcare needs are unique and change throughout each woman's lifetime.
- We believe that women live in families that are self-defined and can include members who are not related by blood or marriage.
- We believe a family-centered philosophy and delivery of maternal newborn care are important in assisting families with the childbearing experience.
- We believe that comprehensive pediatric care addresses the unique developmental needs of each child and her/his family.
- In order to provide sensitive healthcare to women/children/families, we believe that our services need to be:
  - Caring, competent, and offered in a professional manner that emphasizes respect for individuals.
  - Nondiscriminatory and without financial, racial, or cultural bias.
  - Safe, cost-effective, environmentally aware, and responsible.
  - Wellness oriented, providing lifelong educational services for both professionals and community.
  - Progressive, dynamic, and ever evolving through continual evaluation of care, outcomes, and community needs.
  - Challenging, satisfying, and professionally rewarding for healthcare providers.
  - Provided in a partnership between healthcare providers and families.

The Good Samaritan Hospital
4th and Walnut Streets
Lebanon, PA 17042

The Vernon and Doris Bishop Maternal Healthcare Center
"New Beginnings Birth Series"
191-bed hospital
Level I SRMC Maternity Service
Level I Newborn Service
13 LDRPs

- Conversion of a conventional obstetrics program to SRMC in 1998.
- 100% nonseparation of mothers and babies.

Some Comments From Mothers

- Mother, age 30, para 1: "I liked having the baby with me a lot. She was so good at night it was no problem at all. Actually, I kept her in bed with me most of the night. The only time she left my room my entire stay was for her weight check on night shift, and they came for her for blood tests. The doctor did her baby exams in my room. I think if she had not been with me I would have worried about her."
- Mother, age 19, para 2: "I liked having the baby in my room a lot better than if they had kept her in the nursery. The nights were not a problem; I loved it. The only time she left my room was for weight check at night, and they took her for blood tests. The doctor did my baby exam right in my room. I think if she had not been with me I would have worried about her."
- Mother, age 23, para 1: "Having the baby with me was wonderful. I just felt good about my whole stay. Someone was always willing to come help me if I needed to spend time in the bathroom. And when she left at night for her half-hour weight check, I really missed her. The doctor examined her in my room one day, and the other time the doctor

came in late at night for a C-section so the nurses took the baby to the doctor in the nursery."

- Mother, age 28, multip: "Having the baby stay with me was fine. Nights were okay and did not create a problem. I had baby with me my whole stay."
- Mother, age 30, para 2: "It was really nice having the baby in the room all the time. I liked it better this way than having the baby in the nursery all the time like my last visit. I just liked being there when he woke up. I am someone he knows rather than a stranger to him. I also thought it was fun to spend time with him alone without visitors there, that way I could hold him and enjoy him when he was awake. Nights were fine. Last time in the hospital, my baby came out to feed on demand so the only difference this time was that I was there when he woke up."
- Mother, age 36, para 2: "I liked having the baby in my room. Except at night it worked best for me to have her go to the nursery. The nurses were flexible. The baby was always checked in the nursery by the doctor."
- Mother, age 30, para 2: "I liked having the baby in the room a lot. One night I did have her go out because she was so fussy. She even spent the day in my room after my tubal and that night too. She is a good baby so it went well. The doctor checked her in my room, but one time he did it in the nursery because that was where she was when he came. I liked when he checked her in the room best because I could talk to him about her. I did have my son there 3 years ago, and I liked this way better."

New Beginning Birth Suites Philosophy of Care

New Beginnings Start Here . . . It is our belief that each family is special in its own way. Our goals are:

- To make your birth experience a joyous occasion.
- To offer the best care available.

- To provide education needed to support you as you adjust to the growth of your family.
- To respect your beliefs while helping to make the most of your expectations.

Memories of each new beginning start here. Thank you for allowing us to share them with you.

Harbor Hospital Center
3001 South Hanover Street
Baltimore, MD 21225

376-bed hospital
Level II SRMC Maternity Service
Level II Newborn Service
16 LDRPs

- Converted conventional multitransfer OB system to SRMC 1996–1997.
- Known for patient-centered care and state-of-the-art facility for maternity care.

Mercy Health Partners
Fairfield Hospital
3000 Mack Road
Fairfield, OH 45014

190-bed hospital
Level II SRMC Maternity Service
Level II Newborn Service
15 LDRPs

- Hospital is 20 years old, but SRMC only began in 1996. Birth volume over 1,000 in a very competitive environment.
- When selecting nursing staff for the new SRMC service, there were 170 applicants for 40 positions. Applicants interviewed were asked to bring their own mission statements.
- Management and administration are committed to SRMC.
- All patient education classes/programs are taught by RNs working in SRMC.

Mission Statement From Catholic Health Partners

The mission of Catholic Health Partners extends the healing ministry of Jesus by improving the health of our communities with emphasis on people who are poor and underserved.

Values

Catholic Health Partners demonstrates behaviors reflecting our core values of compassion, excellence, human dignity, justice, sacredness of life, and service.

Vision Statement for Team Building, Family Birth Center at Fairfield

The mission of the Family Birth Center is to provide optimal family-centered care, while upholding the Mercy values. We ensure a safe, compassionate, and professional atmosphere. We respect the cultural diversity and experiences of individual families and each other. We reflect this by working together in a progressive and supportive environment, responding to the growing need of the community.

Via Christi Regional Medical Center
St. Joseph Campus
3600 E. Harry Street
Wichita, KS 67218

Family Birthplace
412 (staffed)-bed hospital
Level II SRMC Maternity Service
Level II Newborn Service
20 LDRPs

Family Birthplace Philosophy

The departmental philosophy is consistent with the philosophy of the Medical Center and the Patient Care Services Division of the Medical Center.

The employees of the Family Birthplace believe:

- The family unit serves as the primary functional and structural unit of belonging. The health and well-being of the individual is a direct reflection of the integrity of the family unit. The family unit may have a broad and varied definition, unique to each person.
- Childbearing is a normal physiologic process of human growth and development. Within this process exists the potential for developmental, maturational, emotional, and physiologic crisis. Crisis within the life cycle can pose internal and external stress and may have a positive or negative effect on future well-being.
- The experience of childbirth is influenced by past experiences and perceptions and likewise has an impact on the future growth and development of the individual, the family, and, ultimately, society as a whole.
- In summary, human behavior and emotions are shaped and influenced by environmental forces; therefore, the department and environment must strive to recognize these philosophical premises and create an environment of dignity, warmth, caring, and safety for the childbearing family.

HOSPITALS WITH 1,500 TO 2,000 BPY

- Elmhurst Memorial Hospital
- Memorial Medical Center, Springfield, IL
- St. Francis Women's and Family Hospital
- Wilcox Women's Pavilion, Legacy Good Samaritan Hospital and Medical Center
- Women's East Pavilion

Elmhurst Memorial Hospital
200 Berteau Avenue
Elmhurst, IL 60126

Family Birthing Center
425-bed hospital
Level II SRMC Maternity Service
Level II Special Care Nursery
26 LDRPs

- The Family Birth Center has a patient satisfaction score of 4.65 on a scale of 5.
- A large portion of program emphasis and dollars is on education to new parents. "We decided against the dinners and gift baskets because we believe the greatest gift we can give is education, which is a gift that lasts a lifetime. We distribute the reference book *Caring for Your Baby and Young Child— Birth to Age 5* or, for repeat patients, the book *Caring for Your School-Age Child— Ages 5 to 12*. Both books are childcare

books endorsed by the American Academy of Pediatrics. We are considering using *Your Child's Health,* by Barton Schmidt, as well."

- All staff nurses make post-discharge phone calls to "fill in the gaps" of knowledge deficits and boost the confidence of new families.

Philosophy of Care

At Elmhurst Hospital, we believe that:

- Childbirth is a normal life process and one of its most special events.
- A loving, supportive, and safe environment promotes a positive childbirth experience.
- Knowledge and support are the keys to a successful transition to parenthood.
- Family involvement is an integral part of the childbirth experience.

Memorial Medical Center
701 North First
Springfield, IL 62781-0001

500-bed hospital
Level II SRMC Maternity Service
Level II Newborn Service
18 LDRPs

- Known in the community for quality nursing care, family friendly, flexibility in care of families, and superior education program for new parents and families.
- All staff have an area of "expert" skills (labor or nursery/Level II nursery), plus all staff are cross-trained to mother–baby care.
- The program boosted obstetrics' market share steadily from an all-time low of 30% in 1990 to 49% in 1997. Births increased 40% during the same period. Since the unit's inception, managed care contracts have become a reality, and we believe that positive feelings about the SRMC program have helped attract some of these contracts.
- A recent employee satisfaction survey conducted on the new family maternity suites showed nurses were pleased with the change to SRMC. This is a significant success, given the tremendous turbulence the staff went through.

- Staff nurses continue to grow in their expanded roles, and the unit-based council provides guidance for ongoing improvement in knowledge and skills.

St. Francis Women's and Family Hospital
125 Commonwealth Drive
Greenville, SC 29615

319-bed hospital
Level II SRMC Maternity Service
Level II Newborn Service
24 LDRPs

- 100% cross-trained LDRP staff provides mother–baby/couplet care. A small number of babies are sent to the nursery at night, but an LDRP nurse provides care in the nursery.

Hospital Mission Statement

We are a community of women and men dedicated to continuing the healing ministry of Jesus. We strive for excellence in providing service to all who need us.

We are energized by an atmosphere of joy, mutual respect, and compassion to find better ways of serving.

Service Line Mission Statement

Women's and Children's Services will be a vital and integral piece of the St. Francis Health System. We will serve the women and children of the Upstate, providing exceptional care by using the strengths of each employee.

Shared Values

Compassion. We demonstrate a caring manner and respect the dignity of all.
Competence. We provide quality services and perform our duties as capably as possible.
Collaboration. We work together in a spirit of mutual support as we carry out our mission.
Creativity. We strive to find better ways to serve.

Vision

To provide a lifetime of compassionate, quality healthcare to all those we serve in the Greenville area by offering a continuum of integrated services that will enhance the health status of our community.

- Provide the highest quality, most cost-effective healthcare possible
- Value the dignity of our patients, our employees, and our physicians
- Ensure that our comprehensive healthcare services include the highest degree of compassion and comfort
- Empower our employees to work as a team in creating the kind of environment that enhances the healing process
- Consistently develop and improve ourselves personally and professionally
- Continuously improve planning operations and service delivery
- Listen—to our patients, our employees, our physicians, and the community we serve—as we meet their needs and expectations

Wilcox Women's Pavilion
Legacy Good Samaritan Hospital and Medical
  Center
1015 NW 22nd Avenue
Portland, OR 97210

279-bed hospital
Level III SRMC Maternity Service
Level I Newborn Service
23 LDRPs

- Listed in *Self* magazine's "America's 10 Best Hospitals When You Are Having a Baby" (December 1996).
- High rate of customer satisfaction.
- Tenured nursing staff.
- The average years of service for nurses on the Wilcox Women's Pavilion at Legacy Good Samaritan Hospital is 17 years.
- The staff has a strong commitment to providing excellent care to our patients and families.
- Cross-training took about 3 years. It was interesting that about 2½ years after the move to LDRPs, there was an obvious change in the unit staff. The nursing and medical staff had developed more comfort

and confidence in their roles and were referring to each other in their old area of expertise less often.
- The SRMC facility was opened in February of 1991. It was exciting to watch staff discover they could learn new skills and not only become competent, but experts in new areas. They also grew in their ability to cope with other changes in the healthcare environment.
- Staff continues to gravitate to their areas of preference in perinatal nursing; however, some of the staff have come to love new areas.

Legacy Women's & Children's Services—Vision

To create a culture of excellence in a community of caring.

Legacy Women's & Children's Services—Mission

The Women's and Children's Division builds on the strong foundation of Legacy Health System, striving for excellence in all of our endeavors. As the regional leader in comprehensive care for women and children of all ages, we value strong and effective working relationships, including those with our community partners.

- Our patients and their families come first with us. We are sensitive to the impact of our communications and actions on them. Each of us is responsible for understanding the needs of our patients, and actively partnering with them in developing solutions. We support and hold each other accountable for the responsibility and privilege of providing care. We promote an enriching work setting that fosters professionalism, participation, and ongoing learning.
- Dedication and passion for excellence are values of all of our teams. We provide the highest quality of clinical care for women and children, concentrating on technical expertise and creativity in meeting physical, educational, psychosocial, and spiritual needs. Enhancing quality is the purpose of all

of our efforts, incorporating best practices, managing with data, and effectively managing resources.

- We hold ourselves to the highest standards of respect and compassion for others, acknowledging and embracing diversity. We focus on family integration, and do so in an environment sensitive to individual needs.

Women's East Pavilion
1751 Gunbarrel Road
Chattanooga, TN 37421

Freestanding 28-bed Women's Pavilion
Level II SRMC Maternity Service
Level IIA Newborn Service
16 LDRPs

- 98% patient satisfaction rate.
- Rapid growth to one third of OB market share.
- 100% of babies are with their mothers both day and night.
- Women's East Pavilion is a full-service, 28-bed, 24-hour, inpatient/outpatient hospital that delivers patient-focused, wellness-oriented, family-centered care.
- It is a facility in which both women and the healing professionals share the role of medical care and a commitment to education as the foundation of wellness.
- Women's East Pavilion has 16 family birthing suites dedicated to the care of the expectant family. All patient care, from admission through discharge, takes place in a single room.
- The service is dedicated to family-centered care and educating the low-risk expectant and/or newly born family.
- Nursing care is provided through highly skilled registered nurses who have at least 3 years of training in labor and delivery and have had cross-training in mother–baby care. Patient care partners (nursing assistants) support the care team in a multidimensional role.
- It is the goal of Women's East Pavilion to minimize the number of personnel with whom the patient interacts, providing increased continuity of patient care and education.

- Anesthesia services are provided around the clock with a dedicated operating room conveniently located on the same level as the maternity care unit.
- The level II nursery provides stabilization and transitional care for the sick newborn. Care is provided by neonatal nurse practitioners who work in-house around the clock with neonatologist support.
- The Parents Inn, a room dedicated to families of infants confined to the nursery after the mother's discharge, provides convenient access for neonatal care and breastfeeding. Transport teams are available to assist when needed for high-risk mothers and neonatal emergencies.

Women's Services

- The Women's Services Unit is a 12-bed nursing unit dedicated to the medical and surgical care of women. Staff in this unit encourage patient-involved and family-centered care. Patients are received through direct admits.
- Women are commonly admitted for such low-risk procedures as PID, abdominal and vaginal hysterectomies, and bladder repair.
- The care team, comprised of experienced registered nurses, places emphasis on pre-op and post-op teaching to facilitate recovery and ongoing education to prepare the patient for self-care at home.
- Cesarean birth families return to this unit for care that is directed to meet the specialized needs of operative birth.

Women's Resource Center

- The Women's Resource Center serves as a central point of educational resources for women of the Chattanooga area, including but not limited to those women who are patients of Women's East Pavilion. Programming is centered on the life cycle of women from premenstrual age to the senior years. The Director of Pavilion Resources is a registered nurse with a background in education and counseling.
- The goal of the center is to work with the patient from the initial entry into the health-

care system through discharge and beyond. Programming is planned according to population needs and interests and is provided by experts in the various topic areas.

- Services for the Women's Resource Center include: childbirth education programs, including early pregnancy, sibling and post-partum classes; the lactation station, a full-service breastfeeding support and counseling program that also provides access to pump rental; a resource lending library; community seminars; counseling; and case management for inpatients.

Core Values

Patient centered
　　Family oriented
　　Personalized
Holistic caring
　　Wellness
Innovative
　　Unique
　　State of the art
Inclusive
　　Knowledgeable
　　Comprehensive
　　Accessible
　　Racially and ethnically diverse
Stewardship
　　Fiscally responsible
　　Cost-effective

Mission

Women's East Pavilion, inspired by the healing missions of Erlanger Medical Center and Memorial Hospital, is committed to providing quality, effective, patient-focused, family-oriented care for women.

HOSPITALS WITH 2,000 TO 3,000 BPY

- The Birthplace at Gaston Memorial Hospital
- Medical Center of Central Georgia
- St. Mary's Medical Center
- Waukesha Memorial Hospital, Inc.

The Birthplace at Gaston Memorial Hospital
2525 Court Drive
Gastonia, NC 28053

470-bed hospital
Level II SRMC Maternity Service
Level II–III Newborn Service
23 LDRPs

- Payer mix improvements began in Women's Program and spread to rest of facility.
- All nursing staff provide mother–baby care; 60% provide labor and birth plus mother–baby care; 40% provide mother–baby and nursery care.

Women's Health Mission Statement

We value the knowledge that promotes women's health and wellness and strive to continually educate ourselves and our patients on these issues.

We respect the importance of the family and encourage family involvement and support in our patients' lives.

We recognize birth to be a unique, individual, and natural process and provide competent and caring staff to support mother, child, and family during this joyful event.

Medical Center of Central Georgia
777 Hemlock Street
Macon, GA 31201

Family Birth Center
518-bed hospital
Level III SRMC Maternity Service
Level III Newborn Service
21 LDRPs
80% of mother–baby staff is cross-trained to labor and delivery, and vice versa.

Family Birth Center—Philosophy

We believe childbirth is one of life's most celebrated events, and, to this end, we recognize the importance of family unity.

We believe in and respect a woman's individuality and the right to make choices.

Therefore, our Family Birth Center staff is dedicated to providing families with a supportive and personalized childbirth experience by practicing family-centered maternity care.

Family Birth Center—Mission

We support the hospital's mission, vision, and values by providing the highest quality family-centered maternity care:

- With compassion, respect, and dignity for each individual without bias
- In a timely manner that best meets the individualized needs of our clients
- Coordinated through interdisciplinary team collaboration to ensure continuity and seamless delivery of care to the greatest extent possible
- In a manner that maximizes the efficient use of our financial and human resources by streamlining our processes, decentralizing services, altering provider roles, enhancing communications, continuing staff education, and ensuring technological enhancement.

St. Mary's Medical Center
901 45th Street
West Palm Beach, FL 33407

433-bed hospital
Level III SRMC Maternity Service
Level III Newborn Service
3 separate units: 2 of 16 LDRPs; 1 of 10 LDRPs

- High percentage of mothers keeping babies in room 24 hours.
- Conversion of a conventional multitransfer obstetrics service to SRMC occurred over 10 years ago.

Philosophy of the Perinatal Unit

We believe that pregnancy and childbirth demand physical, social, and psychological adaptation to individuals and families. Adaptation, in large part, depends on a family's ability to perceive stress realistically and to use adequate coping mechanisms to reduce and adapt to that stress.

New families are vulnerable during this transition period and require assistance in strengthening inner resources to enable them to cope with these stresses, and to learn to parent.

We believe that the childbearing family must be supported, not controlled, during the birthing process, in order for them to achieve a positive perception of the birth experience.

We acknowledge childbirth as a major event in people's lives, and in the most important institution in our society—the family.

We, the Maternal/Child staff at St. Mary's hospital, focus our care on the family as a unit—while maintaining the physical safety of all.

It is our commitment to assist, counsel, and care for the expectant mothers, fathers and their families, and to share with them the wonder of the birthing process. We believe that the patient, her family, and others who are significant in her life have the right to certain expectations about childbirth, and to have these expectations fulfilled.

We emphasize the normal, natural aspects of the creative event of childbirth, and we utilize practices that focus on family needs. We treat each family as individuals, with dignity and respect; we administer safe, effective, and sensitive care to them. This compassion and concern for family needs revolve around a holistic person-centered perspective.

Increased continuity to the family is achieved with the planning and evaluation of care by a professional team of nurses who have continuous accountability for the family from admission to discharge; through labor, delivery, and the postpartum recuperation of the family.

Our goal is to offer our support so a new family can begin.

Waukesha Memorial Hospital, Inc.
725 American Avenue
Waukesha, WI 53188-5099

280-bed hospital
Level III SRMC Maternity Service
Level III Newborn Service
30 LDRPs

- Hospital best known for tertiary services: NICU, perinatology, and SRMC family-focused care.
- Key findings of recent patient focus groups: most important factor in choosing a hospital was SRMC and NICU.

- Evergreen Hospital Medical Center
- Pomona Valley Hospital Medical Center
- Shawnee Mission Medical Center, Saint Luke's Shawnee Mission Health System
- St. John's Hospital and Medical Center
- Wellstar Family Birthplace, Cobb Hospital

Evergreen Hospital Medical Center
12040 NE 128th Street
Kirkland, WA 98034

"Family Maternity Center"
149-bed hospital
Level III SRMC Maternity Service
Level II Newborn Service
36 LDRPs, designed in three clusters of 12 LDRPs in each cluster

- Listed in *Self* magazine's "America's 10 Best Hospitals When You Are Having a Baby" (December 1996).

Evolution and Structure of Evergreen's Family Maternity Center—Development of a Comprehensive Perinatal Program

Evolution

1972—Conventional obstetric program (hospital opened)
1984—Beginning plans to move from a medical model to an educational model of care
1985—Developed a written philosophy of care and practiced single-room maternity care in our newly remodeled unit
1992—Opened a new 36-bed LDRP unit (three clusters of 12 LDRPs each)
1996—Midwives in practice with physicians

Current Program Structure

Family maternity education
    Classes
Pondering parenthood to transition to parenthood
Baby parent classes
Mother-to-mother volunteers—promotes interdependence (help and cooperate with each other to grow into parenthood)

Family maternity center—single-room maternity care
    Shared governance teams
        Family-centered maternity care (FCMC) leadership team
        FCMC staffing committee
        FCMC professional practice committee (includes QA)
        FCMC team building committee
        FCMC/SCN charge nurses
    Nursing leadership is encouraged to attend physician section meetings
Special care nursery (level 2)
    Boarding program
    Care conferences
    Parent support group meets once a week
    Case management
    Home phototherapy
Maternal fetal medicine (perinatology)
    High-risk pregnancy
    Genetic counseling
    Antepartum testing
    Diabetic teaching
Breastfeeding center
    Baby-friendly hospital initiative—first baby-friendly hospital in the country
    Supporting and educating staff and families about the ten steps to successful breastfeeding
    Outpatient clinic
    Telephone resource
    Inpatient and SCN rounds in morning and evening
    Inpatient class—bath and baby care given twice each day
Postpartum care center
    Physical examination of mother and infant, nutritional assessment, and a feeding evaluation
    Care planning
    Outcome data
    97% of moms and babies seen at 3 to 4 days postpartum
Family maternity center professional education program
    Coursework in breastfeeding
    Preceptor program
    Consulting on single-room maternity care
    Medical conference focusing on clinical issues

Nursing staff 100% cross-trained to mother–baby care

95% of nursing staff cross-trained to labor and birth care

Separate level II nursery staff who also provide mother—baby care

Continuous Value Improvement

Utilize process improvement teams—multidisciplinary teams from the hospital, provider office staff, and patients.

Decrease cost per delivery—control dollars through changing practice. Manage care and you manage cost:

- Inductions
- Epidurals
- Cesarean section rate
- LOS—in hours
- Supplies
- Overhead expenses
- Staffing

Develop a focused process of coordinated communication of what maternity patients can expect within our medically safe, cost-effective family maternity length-of-stay package.

- Look at how the birth relates to the whole continuum of care (a speed bump in the road of perinatal care).
- Includes a three-part registration form the patient fills out in the office; two copies are sent to the hospital admitting department.
- "The Maternity Patient Information Guide"—given to the patient in the provider's office at 12 weeks of pregnancy.
  - A consistent message given to the patient in all written information: *Pregnancy, Childbirth and the Newborn,* "The Maternity Patient Information Guide," "The Mother and Baby Care Booklet," and "Your Baby in the Special Care Nursery."

All caregivers participate in an extended family maternity pathway, which includes all clinical services from inpatient hospital registration to the postpartum care center visit.

Evergreen Family Maternity Center Philosophy

We believe that:

- Birth is one of life's most special events.
- Birth and parenting occur with greater ease, comfort, and joy when parents assume their roles with knowledge.
- Birth is a natural, physiologic process that can be a positive time of growth.
- Parents can make decisions and accept responsibility for their own healthcare.
- Family, visitors, nurses, physicians, midwives, and all hospital personnel are regarded with dignity and respect.

Pomona Valley Hospital Medical Center
1798 North Garey Avenue
Pomona, CA 91767

The Women's Center
398-bed hospital
Level II SRMC Maternity Service
Level II Newborn Service
48 LDRPs
Converted a traditional multitransfer obstetrics service to SRMC in 1992.

Philosophy of Care—The Women's Center

- Family centered
- Each family is unique in its needs and background. Care is individualized to meet the unique cultural, spiritual, emotional, and physical needs of the mother, infant, and family.
- The mother determines who her family is.
- 100% of babies are with their mothers during the day.
- 80% to 90% of babies are with their mothers at night.

Scope of Services

Prenatal education
Lamaze/teen Lamaze
Baby care basics
Sibling preparation

VBAC class
Infant/child CPR
Breastfeeding
Cesarean birth class
Great beginnings
CPSP
Therapeutic
Delivery
High-risk delivery
Transport programs
Inpatient antepartum
Triage
NICU, level II with surgical center designation
Diabetic care
Postnatal education and support—home
Baby assessment
ADL assistance
Lactation consultation
Mom assessment
Antibody therapy
Ongoing support
Cancer
Menopause
Genetic counseling
Women's health fairs
Grandparenting
Babysitter classes
Lactation visits (phone)
Parenting classes
Boot camp for dads

Nursing Satisfaction—Single-Room Maternity Care

- 100 nurses cross-trained in 6 years
- Merged three nursing units, less "We" versus "They"
- Less fragmentation of care
- Improved standards of practice, skills, flexibility
- Increased ownership, pride, morale
- Waiting list for transfers to SRMC
- Low turnover rate

Improved Clinical Outcomes—Single-Room Maternity Care

- Comprehensive cross-training program
- Increased education, questioning, growth of staff
- Improved assessment skills
- Improved standards of care/practice
- Multidisciplinary approach to care
- Reduction of patient complications, poor outcomes
- Quality of care improved with cross-trained nursing staff
- Active management of labor with ambulation, physiologic positioning, and use of Jacuzzi tub

Physician Satisfaction—Single-Room Maternity Care

- Improved physician satisfaction with nursing care
- Collaborative practice, trusting relationship
- Comprehensive perinatal-neonatal services reassuring to physicians
- Physician associate liaison program

Patient Satisfaction—Single-Room Maternity Care

Customer satisfaction team: Members from SRMC nursing staff, manager, marketing, previous patient

- Review patient satisfaction surveys
- Follow-up phone calls
- Problem resolution
- Feedback to nursing staff, obstetricians, and pediatricians
- Customer satisfaction high
- In Press Ganey surveys, 93% recommending hospital

Financial Outcomes—Single-Room Maternity Care

- Flexible staffing
- Flexible hours for peak census
- Reduced hours per patient day
- Reduced overall cost
- Cross-trained staff for maximum flexibility

Requirements for Staff

The maternity services staff consists of registered nurses, licensed vocational nurses, certified nursing assistants, obstetric techs, unit secretaries, and RN student nurse extern workers. In addition, but not limited to, the multidisciplinary team consists of medical social workers, respiratory, lab, pharmacy, admitting, family birth service staff, perinatal staff nurses and physicians, OB physicians, CPSP staff, and NICU staff and physicians.

Staffing Guidelines

Staff is assigned to patient care based on their level of competence and the acuity level of the patient population.

Key Elements to Succeed

- Cross-training is number one
- Involving staff members in all decisions
- The "change" is not an option; the "design" to get there is
- Never give up
- The management teams' commitment

Mission

To improve the health status of women, children, and their families by providing comprehensive, high-quality, cost-effective, state-of-the-art healthcare services.

Philosophy of the Women's Center

The Women's Center is designed to be the resource for healthcare, for women and children in the greater Pomona Valley. Its mission is consistent with the mission of Pomona Valley Hospital Medical Center, and is structured upon a family-centered philosophy for the delivery of healthcare services.

Family-Centered Maternity Care Philosophy

I. We believe that the family is the basic unit of society.
II. We believe that each family is unique and different in its needs and background.
III. We believe that women are partners in their healthcare.

IV. We believe that family support and involvement are important in childbearing.
V. We believe that the mother determines who her family is.
VI. We believe that pregnancy and birth are normal events for most women.
VII. We believe that the role of the nurse is to provide support to the family during the time surrounding birth.
VIII. We believe that care should be individualized and address the unique emotional, spiritual, and physical needs of the mother, infant, and family.

**Shawnee Mission Medical Center
Saint Luke's Shawnee Mission Health System
9100 W. 74th Street
Shawnee Mission, KS 66204**

350-bed hospital
Level II SRMC Maternity Service
Level II Newborn Service
18 LDRPs

- "Most preferred" maternity service in Kansas City, according to 1998 NCR Healthcare Market Research.
- Birth volume increases each year.

SMMC Vision for Women and Children's Services

The Shawnee Mission Medical Center's Women and Children's service line is committed to providing a high-quality, customer service driven, comprehensive continuum of women and newborn services, partnering with physicians, other healthcare providers, and payers, that will enable most moms and babies to remain in their community and will positively impact mortality and morbidity rates in Kansas City. We will be a market leader in Kansas City for women and children's services.

**St. John's Hospital and Medical Center
22101 Moross Road
Detroit, MI 48236-2172**

608-bed hospital
Level III SRMC Maternity Service
Level III Newborn Service
31 LDRPs

- Birth volume reached goal.
- Patient satisfaction increased.

Wellstar Family Birthplace
Cobb Hospital
3950 Austell Road
Austell, GA 30127

322-bed hospital
Level III SRMC Maternity Service
Level III Newborn Service
26 LDRPs

- Listed in *Self* magazine's "America's 10 Best Hospitals When You Are Having a Baby" (December 1996).
- Six of these 26 LDRPs were added in 1997 due to volume of growth. The original SRMC facility had 20 LDRPs.

Mother–Baby Couplet Care

- Because we believe families belong together—sometimes needing support and assistance—we have developed "Mother-Baby Couplet" care. This is a progressive concept in which the nurse who cares for mother also cares for baby and interacts with all family members.
- There is no traditional normal newborn nursery.
- Wellstar Family Birthplace's philosophy extends to the whole family. Women are admitted with their families, so there are no restrictions on siblings and grandparents coming and going—unless the mother wants

to set them. Not only is the mom hearing about how to diaper and feed the baby, but the grandparents are as well.

- Everything focuses back on the family and keeping that family unit together. The better we educate the entire family, the better the mother's support system.

Philosophy of the Women's Center

We believe:

- That women should be offered choices for themselves and their children.
- That women are entitled to healthcare with dignity.
- That a positive perinatal experience is an enduring contribution to women.
- That caring is demonstrated by commitment.
- That family unity is best supported by care provided to the mother and her baby by the same nurse.

Therefore we commit ourselves to:

- A service orientation that offers choices to women and their families.
- Supporting the choices women and their families make.
- Providing healthcare with dignity and showing respect for the individual.
- Open communication and teamwork among all perinatal healthcare givers—physicians, nurses, and other staff.
- Continuing medical and nursing education to ensure quality care.
- Recognition of the importance of each member of the healthcare team including the woman herself, physicians, nurses, and other healthcare providers.

Index

References with "t" denote tables; those with "f" denote figures; those with "b" denote boxes